Girl, Get Up

An Inspirational Guide for Women Living with Autoimmune Disease, Chronic Illness and Pain

Whitney L. Brooks, *Visionary Author*

Co-Authored By:
Sonia Austin-Moore, Karell Bailey, Trimika Cooper, Claudia Massey, Lare Ngofa, Treina Owen, Karen Robinson, Chazley Williams

Printed in the United States of America.

ISBN: 979-8-9876649-9-5
Edited, Formatted and Published by Empower Her Publishing, LLC
empowerherpublishing.com

Table of Contents

Introduction

In the labyrinth of life, where adversity lurks around every corner, the voices of women emerge as beacons of resilience, guiding others through the darkest of tunnels. *Girl, Get Up* is more than just a book—it's a roadmap of courage, a testament to the unyielding spirit of women battling autoimmune diseases, chronic illnesses, and the relentless grip of pain.

Within these pages, you will find a tapestry of personal testimonies woven with threads of strength, perseverance, and hope. Each story is a testament to the indomitable will of women who refuse to let illness define their lives. From the shadows of diagnosis to the triumph of acceptance, these women's journeys transcend the confines of suffering, offering inspiration to all who walk a similar path.

Autoimmune diseases and chronic illnesses cast a shadow over the lives of millions of women, each one facing a unique set of challenges. Whether it's the debilitating pain of rheumatoid arthritis, the pervasive path of lupus, sickle cell or diabetes, the recovery after cancer or stroke, or the unpredictable course of ulcerative colitis or premenstrual dysphoric disorder, these conditions test the limits of resilience and resolve. Yet, within the depths of their struggle, women find the courage to rise again, to reclaim their lives with unwavering determination.

Girl, Get Up is a rallying cry for women everywhere, a call to arms against the tyranny of illness and despair. Through the voices of those who have walked this path before, readers will find solace, strength, and solidarity. This book is not just about surviving—it's about thriving in the face of adversity, about embracing the journey with courage and grace.

As you embark on this journey through *Girl, Get Up*, may you find inspiration in the stories of resilience contained within its pages. May you be empowered to face your own challenges with renewed strength and determination. For in the company of these women, you will discover the true meaning of courage—the courage to rise, to reclaim, and to triumph against all odds.

Welcome to *Girl, Get Up*, where the voices of women echo with the power of resilience, and where every story is a testament to the triumph of human perseverance.

Ugghhhhh, Here We Go Again!
Sonia Austin-Moore

"I'm an Introvert, but an Extrovert to whom I want to talk to."

(Nephew) Ryan

I have always stayed to myself. I'm not very social; I don't ask for help, and I don't let anyone know what's going on in my life. I feel safe riding solo, keeping everything to myself. That way, there's no one to judge me or assume they know what I'm going through. To be honest, I'm pretty sure someone out there has gone through everything I have gone through or if not, at least close. Somewhere, someone has the same feelings, emotions, breakdowns, depression, and the list goes on. In fact, I'm pretty sure someone is shaking their head while reading this and saying, "Yep, that's me toooo!" Whelp (hands raised), here's me being an Extrovert. I'm opening up and letting everyone into "my world".

2005

I moved back to Richmond three days before I started the Police Academy and everything's going as well as it could go in the academy. Then, one day,

I was in severe pain. The cramps hit me out of nowhere and to the locker room "WE" went. You're probably wondering "Weeee?" Yes, you go everywhere in pairs. I checked to see what was going on and I was okay. I just took four Advils. Don't judge me. After that day, the cramps were coming more frequently, the pain was increasing, and nothing I did would make it better. Then one day "WE" had to run to the bathroom and I checked myself again. My eyes grew wide and I cursed to myself loudly in my head. I had to double up a sanitary napkin and I was really confused about what was going on. Almost every hour, I found myself asking to go to the bathroom. I was not in pain, but was constantly changing. I didn't want my training Sergeant to think I was trying to get out of training so I had to speak to him. My thought was, "Girlllllll, you can't be embarrassed. You are 34 years old and he's probably in his 40's. He should understand." So the next day I asked him if we could speak in private and I told him what was going on. "My period is very heavy and I'm changing my pad a lot. Can I go to the bathroom when needed?" He looked at me and said, "Okay." Needless to say, my Academy life was the beginning of my first "Ugghhhhh, here we go again!"

2006

I'm in pain and my menstrual is consistently heavier. I'm beginning to think this is normal. I haven't told anyone what's been going on. I've learned to just deal with it. I'll figure out what I need to do and keep it moving. During my one week a month for work, I would stack two long overnight pads in my panties and wear compression shorts under my uniform pants or whatever I wore for the day. As the years went on, it got worse. Those who know me, know I don't sugar coat much of anything, and OMG, I was miserable, absolutely miserable. Soon after, my left side started hurting. Let's put this in perspective: 1) My menstrual is so heavy I'm changing my pads almost hourly, and 2) The pain from my cramps hurt so badly as if someone punched me, and 3) Now I have a left side pain. "Ugghhhhh, here we go again!" So I go to the Doc in the Box (better known as Urgent Care) down the street for my left side pain. I'm basically told they don't see anything wrong and give me some Motrin for the pain. Between the monthly heavy bleeding and the pain on my left side, I swear I should've held stock in Always and Motrin.

2007-2009

Hey y'all, heyyy! Not much has changed. Okay, yeah a lot has changed. I've been to my GYN on several occasions throughout the years because "WE" were all over the internet Googling everything. I was now a certified WebMD Doctor. I do think we all are WebMD Graduates. Nevertheless, "WE" found the answers - fibroids. Yes, those nasty muscular tumors that grow in the wall of the uterus. This apparently was some of the cause of my heavy bleeding, pain, and blood clots, along with endometriosis. Endometriosis is another painful condition, where the inner lining of the uterus grows outside the uterus and the tissue thickens and bleeds every menstrual cycle. The most

3

horrifying thing is, I was now bleeding every month, every day, except for the six days of my cycle. Apparently the lining of my uterus was shedding. "Ugghhhhh, here we go again!"

2009

My family and I went on a family vacation to Florida. What should've been an amazing time turned out to be a miserable experience for me. One highlight, though, was being able to find jean shorts that fit like compression shorts. My trips to the parks consisted of carrying a bag with those overnight long pads with wings, the 20+ pack ones, Motrin and bottled waters. I wore the two pads, compression shorts, and my new fitted jean shorts daily. I'm telling you, I did not have fun on this vacation. Our family photos may seem like I did, but that was for the kids' sake. I slept with a towel under me every night, because each morning I didn't know what to expect. As a woman, if you know how horrible that one week a month is while on your cycle and on vacation that you can't do much of anything, then imagine about 26 days. I know many are probably saying, "Girl, why didn't you use a tampon?" All I can say is, I couldn't. About two days into vacation, I called my doctor in tears. I told her what was going on and asked what I could do. I'm usually a strong person; I don't cry much about anything, but geesh, this was ridiculous. My doctor sent me a prescription of Tamoxifen for a few days and told me that I couldn't take anymore once it was done. By this point, I didn't know if I needed to ration these few pills or take as prescribed. I popped the pills, which cut the bleeding in half. I was down to one pad and I enjoyed the rest of the vacation.

Back from vacation and "Ugghhhhh, here we go again!" The bleeding is back. I immediately called my doctor's office.   Thankfully, I got a same-day appointment and I guess I'm lucky because I work in the city so it didn't take me long to get to my appointment. I let my Sergeant know I had to take a few hours of vacation to run an errand. My doctor was on vacation, so I saw the other doctor who was working in the office. He looked at my huge folder, then looked at me, read a few things and said, "the nurse will come and get you in a few minutes." That's strange, I thought. He didn't push my stomach, ask me any questions, nada. I hopped off the table and went to his office. He asked me to shut the door and slid a pamphlet to me. I looked at him and he said, "I need you to go home and read this (Uterine Cancer Pamphlet), then set up an appointment for surgery. You have cancer." Wait, what? In my mind, the only thing I could say to myself was, "Damn, his bedside manners are frik'n horrible," and then "Sonny, walk out with your head high, like nothing just happened." I said okay to him, grabbed a prescription (Tamoxifen), walked out the office shaking. I anxiously waited for the young lady to slide the glass window to let her know I would call back later for an appointment. I went to my car and cried. After speaking to the one person who knew what was going on, they advised me to wait until my doctor came back from vacation. Then I went back to work and casually picked up where I left off a few hours earlier.

2011

I definitely waited for my doctor to come back. Yes, I had pre-cancerous cells, but my doctor and I agreed we were going to do everything we could first. No surgery. Truthfully, I was tired of the doctor visits and different medicines. I low-key wanted a hysterectomy, but I understood what my doctor was trying to do. Plus, who wants to go into menopause at 40? So here were my options: Endometrial Ablation or Uterine Artery Embolization. I asked two good friends who had the Ablation the pros/cons and they both said they haven't had a menstrual since the procedure. Someone else attested to having minor issues. I opted for the UAE and knew it would last two years. The procedure involved a small cut at the top of my leg near my pelvis followed by a catheter insertion into the artery in my leg. The catheter goes to the arteries that supply the blood to the uterus. They put these small ball things, like a particle, through the catheter and it blocks the blood supply to the fibroids. I was awake the entire time.

2014

Guess what? My left side still hurts and I'm continuously being told nothing is wrong. Guess what else? I started bleeding again. "Ugghhhhh, here we go again!" I made an appointment for the upcoming Monday. Quick exam? Nope - biopsy.

Ouch! The follow-up appointment was made for the next Monday. I went alone, because 1. I'm good, 2. I was putting my foot down and asking for a hysterectomy, and 3. I wasn't leaving without an appointment for surgery. Unfortunately, my appointment didn't go as planned. I was told the cancer cells grew in size and number and I needed to make an appointment the same week for surgery. I then had another biopsy, but it wasn't the same. It hurt so bad that I was sweating and crying. My doctor stopped immediately and just hugged on me while wiping away my tears and sweat. Once I got my life together, I didn't make an appointment, I let the front desk know I would call back in a few days. I'm a mom, so I needed to make sure none of the kids had games, doctors' appointments, or that I didn't have court for work. Why are we like this? I couldn't wait to make it to my car to cry. I had a few more biopsies, a small procedure in the hospital, and a quick family trip to the beach two days before my surgery. Finally, I had a partial hysterectomy, leaving one ovary behind.

2014-2017

My left side hurts and I see bruising and a bulge again. So I took pictures. I am so tired of doctors not believing me. My Doc in the Box doctor definitely thought I was crazy because I overheard her say while she was doing her transcription that nothing was wrong with me. Insert the eye roll I gave her behind the curtain. The doctor gave me a referral to a gastrointestinal doctor. My dad always told me I can fire doctors if I don't feel I am being treated right. Needless to say, after years of being my Doc in the Box, I fired her. The next day, my gastro doctor asked what was wrong and I showed him my pictures. He pushed my stomach a few times and said, "You have either Diverticulitis, Ulcerative Colitis, or Crohn's Disease." Well, I have Ulcerative Colitis and the bulge I would see over the years was my intestines pushing through my stomach wall. Unfortunately, I couldn't afford my medicine. I used my WebMD Degree and researched as if I was trying to get my PhD. I did an allergy test, stopped eating the foods I was allergic to, and continued working out. I found that by working out, my flare ups went from about ten a year to two a year.

2018

I texted my friend to let her know I wasn't going out one night because I was feeling *weird*. I always wake up early, but this time it was around 9 am or 10 am when a coworker called and said I sounded like I was asleep. "No, I'm wide awake," I told her. After we spoke, my left hand started tingling. My mom said, "Sonny, you probably slept on it wrong." I knew I hadn't, but I went to the room to watch TV in an attempt to carry on with my day. Shortly after, however, my left eye went blurry. I figured it was my new glasses. Then I had chest pain followed by clammy skin and sweating without sweating. Lawd, am I having a heart attack? I got in the shower and hyperventilated. So I stepped out, but lost my balance. My left leg went numb and I became scared.

"Ugghhhhh, here we go again!" I let my daughter know that I was going to run to the doctor real quick. By real quick, I thought it would be a few hours in the ER, but we know how that went. I told my daughter that if I wasn't back before her competition that I would get her a ride. I was feeling better, so I drove myself to the hospital. Do not do this. And yes, I was yelled at, but I also spoke with one of my best guy friends all the way there. When I got to the ER, I felt fine and I spoke with the doctor. He had me perform a few routine tasks like walking to the door and back to him while answering questions. "Who's the President? What's the date? etc." The second time I struggled with the answers. He also had me put my arms in front of me and close my eyes. My left arm would drop and he said it was drifting. Eventually, I had many scans, spoke to a neurologist in Atlanta via video and he asked if I could give permission to receive TPA, a drug used to break up a blood clot and restore the flow of blood to the brain. Once I was released from ICU, I went to an outpatient rehab facility. The strength test showed I had 18% strength on my left side and 99% on my right. I tear up reflecting on this because two days prior, I had just finished a two-a-day in the gym, which I was doing four to five times a week. Then, somehow, in a matter of days, I ended up in a rehab facility building up strength to do simple, everyday things again. I love to nap, but I was sleeping like a newborn baby. Moreover, I was unable to do easy tasks such as twisting the cap on a water bottle or walking around the nurse's station. This is the moment I really cried and became depressed.

2023

I'm still an Introvert. This is hard letting everyone in. Despite my health challenges, I never let any of them define who I am. Someone once told me I was dealt a shitty hand. No, the hand I was dealt helped me learn about myself, my strengths and forced me to not view any setbacks as permanent. I hope after reading this, someone can say "I'm not alone" and in 2024 and beyond, no more "Ugghhhhh, here we go again!"

Dedication

Thank you to my family and friends and everyone who reads my story and finds themselves somewhere within these pages. And thank you to my Smith Crew for yelling to me 15 years ago, "Do you want to join us?" Otherwise, I would probably still be sitting solo to this day.

Sonia Austin-Moore is a mom of three adult children and a grandmother of one. She is an 18-year Veteran with the Richmond Police Department, where for the last 12 of those years she has served as a Forensic Detective. She is also an Adjunct Professor at North Carolina Agricultural and

Technical State University in the Criminal Justice Department. Sonia holds a Master's Degree from Arizona State University in Criminal Justice with Forensics Studies. She is an athlete at heart, and for five seasons, played for the Richmond Black Widows, a Women's Professional Football Team in the WFA League (Full Pads/Tackle). Sonia also joined an African-American Female Powerlifting team where she placed 1st in her age group in two separate deadlift competitions. Sonia is also a proud member of Iota Phi Lambda Sorority, Incorporated, Zeta Rho Chapter, in Petersburg, Virginia.

Thank You to My Pre-Order Supporters!

Donovan Moore

Steven Powell, Sr.

Chloe Crowder

Lin Tyler

Carl Scott

Carlos B

Ronetta Lewis

Dee Dee Anderson
Instagram: @612dna

Kat OConnell

Moise Bonheur
Facebook: @Moisetopaz
Instagram: @Moisetopaz

Crystal Starks-Williams

Ernest Wilford

Willie Ruffin

Afya Njema Fitness LLC

https://linktr.ee/afyanjemafit

Instagram: @Afya_Njema_Fit

Antonia Saunders

Christians Crusaderz, LLC

Facebook:
https://www.facebook.com/christianscrusaderz?mibextid=ZbWKwL

Instagram: @christianscrusaderzllc

LinkedIn: https://www.linkedin.com/in/antonia-saunders-30b342123?utm_source=share&utm_campaign=share_via&utm_content=profile&utm_medium=android_app

Angela Greenidge

Symmion Moore

symmionmoore.wordpress.com

Alexandra Yugga

Telicia Whitehead

Shreekk Crawford

Facebook: Shreekk Crawford

Instagram: @C_Rock99

The Unexpected Struggle
Karell Bailey

"For our present troubles are small and won't last very long. Yet they produce for us a glory that vastly outweighs them and will last forever. So, we don't look at the troubles we can see now; rather, we fix our gaze on things that cannot be seen. For the things we see now will soon be gone, but the things we cannot see will last forever."

Corinthians 4:17-18

I had no idea what 2020 had in store for me. It started off as a typical new year wrapping up holiday travel visiting family. Then the pandemic hit, and like everyone, I found myself balancing working from home and homeschooling my children. Little did I know, this was only the beginning of sorrows for the year.

Once the sticker shock of quarantined life wore off, I thought I had settled into a balanced routine. The boys and I were getting our work done, exercising, and finding fun things to do at home. June rolled in and I noticed I was not feeling my best. I felt a strange, unfamiliar kind of exhaustion. I would get up, fix breakfast for the boys, and immediately need to lay back down because I felt tired and weak. Within a few weeks, a burning pain started in my right breast and armpit. After a self-examination, I discovered a lump about the size of the palm of my hand in my armpit. I convinced myself it was nothing, but that I'd still better be safe and get it checked out. Within two months, I learned that this was indeed something.

My PCP was very encouraging and supportive in the preliminary stages of this process. He moved swiftly, pulling strings to get me seen immediately by specialists to see what was going on. His hope was that it was a minor cyst that could be removed with no further issues or concerns. Unfortunately, the breast cancer specialist he referred me to was not convinced I had a cyst.

Moving with a similar sense of urgency, she scheduled an ultrasound, mammogram, and biopsy. The results came back within a few days, and she reported, "we have ruled out breast cancer, but we cannot rule out other cancers." Excuse me, what? You think I may have cancer? Before I let my mind run too far away, I decided to remain calm until we knew more. There was still a chance it was nothing.

In early August, one day after my 41st birthday, I was in the OR getting prepared for diagnostic surgery. I do not remember much from the day, but I remember waking up groggy and overhearing the doctor tell my husband that as soon as she opened me up, she could see I had Hodgkin's Lymphoma Cancer. She also said that it was everywhere on my right side and in my chest wall. We would wait for pathology to confirm but she was confident in the diagnosis. Within two weeks the diagnosis was confirmed: I had cancer!

I could not believe it. I struggled to process this news. All I could do was cry. So many questions, fears, and emotions hit me all at once and really, ALL I could do was cry. My husband, mother, and sister reassured me I would get through this and be ok. I genuinely believed them, but still, I cried. I was crying, not because this was happening to me, but because I did not want to experience this fight. I did not want God to HAVE TO show up for me in this way. There are so many other people with far greater needs than me, and I did not want Him to take away from them to deal with this thing for me. Nevertheless, here I was reluctantly preparing for one of the hardest battles of my lifetime.

As we began the staging and treatment process, my oncologist shared that she believed my diagnosis was incomplete. Turns out the type of Hodgkin's

Lymphoma I had was a rare, slow growing cancer. The CT and PET scans, however, showed I had both a slow growing lymphoma and a more aggressive fast-growing cancer. Off to UVA Hospital she sent me to see more specialists to receive a full diagnosis.

The lymphoma team started reviewing my case before I arrived. They confirmed my Hodgkin's Lymphoma diagnosis and confirmed I also had a more aggressive Non-Hodgkin's Lymphoma. My mind was reeling! I had not one, but two cancers! I immediately felt like I was drowning and choking at the same time. I tried to remain calm and composed so I could retain everything the doctor said. We were still in a pandemic, so I attended the visit alone. I tried very hard to remember all the tiny details so that I could share with my husband and family. With my full diagnosis confirmed, it was clear a less invasive radiation treatment was off the table and a more aggressive chemo and immunotherapy treatment were the only options for the best chance at remission.

There was no time to waste! No time to sit with my emotions and process the information. We had to get moving so I could start treatment. More appointments, labs, and then off to another OR to have my port installed. No time to heal or grieve over what was happening because it was time for my first treatment within two days of surgery.

Family and friends tried to encourage me with well wishes and prayers. Some even said that if you could have any cancer this was the one to have because it was the "easy cancer". Let me tell you, my cancer experience was anything but "easy". My treatment was a full-day experience. I arrived at 8 am and was there until about 5:30 pm. Treatment Day started with blood work then off to the infusion room for premedication and treatment. My treatment was called RCHOP. It consisted of an immunotherapy drug (Rituxan), three different chemotherapy drugs, and prednisone. At the end of the treatment day the nurse would put an injection patch on me that would administer a shot within 24 hours to help my body begin to regenerate white blood cells. We decided to place the patch on my stomach so that it was less visible to my children. That surprise injection was not something I could ever get used to.

My treatment was a slow process. I was so sensitive to the medications that the nurses had to slow down or stop my infusions several times to check my vitals, let me rest, and allow the side effects to subside. It was brutal! I had several family members and friends call, text, and FaceTime me throughout the day to keep me company and lift my spirits. Thank God for technology! My favorite part of treatment day was seeing my husband and two sons' smiling faces waiting outside to take me home. I was tired and could barely walk but seeing them gave me so much joy.

Beyond the challenges during treatment, I experienced complications and pains during this journey. One complication came eighteen days after my first treatment. I developed pain and itching around my port. A visit to the oncologist and it was only a minor skin infection that should be easily cleared up with antibiotics. Within 48 hours the pain worsened, landing me in the ER. The ER doctor took one look and said my port was infected and would have to be removed immediately! Within the hour, I was rushed off to the OR.

I spent a week in the hospital recovering from the infection. Before going home, a new port was placed on the other side. I transitioned to in-home nurse care for two months to treat the open wound from the removed port. The wound could not be closed to prevent further infections, so I had a gaping hole in my chest! It was a sickening site.

I continued chemotherapy and new side effects popped up. I developed neuropathy (weakness, numbness and pain from nerve damage) in my hands and feet. I wore copper gloves just to pick up things because I could not endure the pain of my skin touching anything. After a month of dealing with the neuropathy, my oncologist lowered one of my chemotherapy drugs to reduce the neuropathy. We were concerned how this would impact treatment but hopeful I was getting enough to still go into remission.

Despite the brutal process, I completed treatment and went into remission. Remission day was a bittersweet day. I was thankful to be in remission but felt extreme guilt for all my husband and family endured during the process. Still, I remained hopeful that I was on the road to recovery and would be back to normal very soon.

I, like most of my loved ones, thought that once I was in remission this ordeal would be over. I expected to have regular checks to make sure I did not relapse. Never did I imagine my body would struggle so badly post-treatment leading to chronic pain.

My oncologist told me it would take 18-24 months for my immune system to rebuild itself. Due to my preexisting asthma, and it still being a pandemic, she required me to stay quarantined long past when the world started opening back up. Once my immune system rebuilt itself, we discovered it did not respond to environmental stimuli the same. Previously, my seasonal allergies would result in the typical allergy symptoms. Now my body responds with a full-on inflammatory response which means excruciating pain throughout my body. The pain feels like my body is compressing on itself.

As if that were not enough to deal with, I started noticing that it was becoming more challenging for me to walk, sit, or get around without assistance. I was diagnosed with early onset arthritis, which is typical for chemo patients. We started pain management treatment, but I was not responding. Then the leg pain and swelling started. After several specialist visits, we discovered I have lymphedema in both legs.

The lymphedema and inflammation are the sources of my daily pain and mobility restrictions. I have twice weekly immunotherapy injections to help calm my immune system and train it to stop having an inflammatory response. The goal is a complete cure, but it is a 3–5-year process to build up my immunity.

Lymphedema and arthritis, however, are not conditions that can be cured. Both ailments will require lifelong management. Twice daily in-home leg compression therapy is currently the best way to manage my condition. Therapy reduces the swelling and leg pain, but there are still many days where I struggle to walk. There are no pain-free days. On the bad days, I still require assistance and care from my husband and family to manage daily tasks. I cannot explain how embarrassing it is to need my husband's help navigating to the bathroom when I am unable to walk on my own. Yes, we vowed in sickness and in health and my husband gladly helps with no complaints. Still, it is disheartening to be almost three years in remission and still require this level of care.

Even more than needing ongoing care, I still have a daily reminder of what I have gone through. I thought post treatment I would "be better" and this would be a distant memory. My reality is that I have no tangible hopes of ever putting this experience in the rearview mirror. So, what keeps me going when I have every reason to let my body quit?

Feel the Pain

I give myself permission to feel my pain. So often we focus on the needs of others because it is easier than dealing with the strain of our situation. I have learned through this process that sometimes I just need to sit with my pain and not push past it. This does not mean I lay and wallow in my pain. Instead, I acknowledge how and what I am feeling. Feeling my pain forces me to listen to my body, be honest about what I need, and take the proper care to get through the day. Becoming more in tune with myself leads to intentionality in communicating my needs to God and others. This is freeing because the guilt and weight of unrealistic expectations are not heaped upon me because I am honest about my daily limits.

Advocate for Myself

While living in constant pain, it is easy to be viewed as a complainer, hypochondriac, or even a weak person. The reality, however, is that no one is living in my skin. Only I know what I am experiencing. Even the most sympathetic caregiver cannot fully understand my struggle. For this reason, I must do what is best for me and be my own advocate. If it does not feel good, or I am not getting better, I keep advocating for myself. I cannot afford to let things build up and become unmanageable because I am staying silent. The squeaky wheel gets the oil! There is help available to ease my pain and suffering. Constant communication and a great medical team makes all the difference.

Go at My Own Pace

The mentally challenging part of living with chronic pain is that I must accept my limitations. Not only physical limitations, but also mental limitations. Some days it takes every bit of brain power just to move. I cannot explain the frustration that I feel to want to run and play with my three children, but my body is unable to respond. Instead of letting my limitations hold me down, I have learned to go at my pace. Ecclesiastes 9:11 reminds me that the race is not given to the swift nor the battle to the strong. Some days my pace is extremely slow and my strength nonexistent. Regardless, I keep going and trust that when I fall short, God's grace is shown to me through others carrying me the rest of the way.

Prayer Support

I would not be here without the prayers of my family and friends. There have been countless days where I wanted to give up. Times where I begged my husband to let me lay down and die. Praise God, somebody prays for me! I am here because on the lowest days and the best days, my loved ones pray for me. I am only as strong as the last prayer prayed for me. I am eternally grateful for my faithful prayer warriors.

The hardest part about living with illness or chronic pain is forcing myself to function "normally" when I feel anything but normal. It would be easy to give up because of my pain. It is a struggle to keep going when I feel weak, but I am reminded in 2 Corinthians 12:9 that God's strength is made perfect in our weakness. This encourages me because there is power in my weakness. That power fuels me to get up, move forward, and fulfill my purpose.

Karell Bailey is a wife and mother of three. She is a native New Yorker with a passion for learning and helping others. Karell and her husband turned their love for children into ministry, spending almost a decade as foster parents for the City of Richmond.

An accountant by profession, Karell has always had a heart for ministry. Surviving lymphoma reminded Karell of how precious life is and encouraged her to take the leap into full-time ministry. Karell strives to live her life in a way that creates memories and makes the places she serves better than when she arrived. She hopes her testimony of pain and endurance will encourage others to keep going when it seems impossible.

Thank You to My Pre-Order Supporters!

Joy Cole

Naomy Rodrigues

Facebook: Nayumes Rodrigues

Instagram: @naoministry

https://www.linkedin.com/in/naomyjrodrigues

Kevin McClatchie

McClatchie Tree & Lawn Care

mcclatchietreeandlawn.com

Facebook: McClatchie Tree & Lawn Care

Natalie Briggs

LaJoy Washington

Simply Sweets by Joy

Simplysweetsbyjoy.com

Facebook: @smiplysweetsbyjoy

Instagram: @simplysweetbyjoy

Daniel Bailey

Cheryl Witherspoon

The Assembly of God's People of the Apostolic
LinkedIn: The Assembly of Gods People of the
Apostolic

Life, and Life More Abundantly
Whitney L. Brooks

It was a beautiful, bright May day, May 13, 2023 to be exact. I eagerly arose that morning, showered, got dressed, even did my makeup, before heading to my office. It was a Saturday, but I was hosting headshots for some of my book publishing clients. Creating author brands is what I do. One by one, the authors arrived for their photo ops. I had scheduled them meticulously in time blocks to ensure everyone's time was maximized, including the photographer's. It was roughly ten of them in total that day and once they had all finished posing and smiling, I indulged in a few shots myself. The camera has always been my friend. I felt so empowered. I took a deep breath, released and headed to pick up my son from my sister's before visiting my mom for a bit. Life was good!

After visiting my mom's for all of a few hours, hee-hee and haha-ing, I announced it's time for Malachi (my handsome little one) and me to leave. I inched forward up off the couch only to be lassoed back into my previous sitting position. That's strange, I thought, but I brushed it off and gave it one more try. Recognizing I did have a full day and it was past my bedtime, I figured I'd put a little more umph into my next attempt to get up off the couch. One hand on the armrest and a little rock back and forth like my Grandma used to do, and that did it - I was up. Though up, my knees were buckling and my ankles felt like they were cracking into little tiny pieces beneath me. I couldn't withstand the weight of my own body. It was too heavy. I had to sit back down. I was fully aware that something was happening in that moment, something I hadn't ever experienced before, and it brought a bit of a chuckle out of me. A chuckle of confusion, I suppose.

Sharing my sentiment, my family also laughed and requested for me to "stop playing around". While I undoubtedly possess a grand sense of humor, this pain I had just experienced in my knees and ankles was far from funny. I took a deep breath, sucked it up, and stood up off the couch again. I needed to make it home and I couldn't sitting on that couch. Each second on my feet felt like blazing fire in my ankles. It burned. It ached. Badly. But I braced myself and took one step at a time towards the door. The struggle intensified putting my shoes on and making it in my car. My legs were beginning to hurt too. By the time I traveled the 10-minute drive from my parents' to my house and attempted to make it out of the car, I wanted to cry. The pain hurt worse with every move. I spent more than 10 minutes sitting in my car in the driveway trying to determine the best way to get out of it and into the house. Thankfully, my son is very patient and he's also so compassionate. At five, he recognized my agony and wanted to assist, but I just knew I couldn't be touched. "I got it, baby," I assured him. "Just give Mommy a second." Eventually, I managed to lift each leg out of the car one at a time and suffer through the pain in my knees and my ankles to get to the door. Now the stairs, I said to myself. I really wanted to crawl, but realized that would require me to use my knees. I was just trying to think of anything that would alleviate the pain in my ankles. They hurt the worst.

Our nighttime routine was probably extended by an hour. I just couldn't get myself together. I didn't know what I had done earlier that day to bring on this kind of pain, but I was on a mental merry-go-round trying to figure it out. I had strutted a little hard in my heels when taking pictures, but that was nothing new. Nothing else I could think of. I figured I should just go to bed and sleep whatever this little episode was off and I'd be brand new the next morning. However, the pain grew more and more excruciating throughout the night. Before I knew it, I couldn't even turn over in the bed. My legs felt like they belonged on a 500-pound man. They were far too heavy for me to lift myself. I didn't have the strength to turn my own body over in the bed. What was happening to me?

As luck would have it, I had to pee, not once, but twice that night. I held it for as long as I could. Anything to keep from getting up on my aching legs, knees, ankles and now feet. My feet hurt so bad, I couldn't put them flat on the floor. I had to walk on the sides of my feet. You know, the walk you do when you've had on heels too long and the bottom of your feet are burning? Except this burning sensation wasn't on the outside of my feet; it was on the inside. After contemplating ways to make it to my bedroom bathroom (just a few feet away) in the least painful way possible, I came up with nothing. At first I thought about crawling again, thinking I would just rather deal with the knee pain than the ankle and feet pain since the ankle and feet pain were worse than the knee pain. But, I realized I wouldn't be able to get up off the floor with this new muscle ache and weakness in my legs now. So...what was I to do? Making it to the bathroom in pain was far better than having to strip the bed, re-make the bed and re-shower in pain from peeing on myself. So again, I took a deep breath, sucked it up, and duck walked to the bathroom. Now for the next challenge: Squatting down to sit on the toilet with aching knees and painful legs. I really did feel like I was being challenged in the boot camp of life and I was failing - miserably!

After giving myself a stern lecture, I vowed to stay in bed and rest all day Sunday. "You've been doing the most, Whitney. Now look at you. Can barely walk.

Can't even make it to the bathroom. You need to sit down somewhere." My body was big mad with me, but rest would do the trick, I thought. Sunday came and I stayed in bed as I promised myself. Well, with the exception of getting up to let the dog out, feeding my son fifty-leven times, getting him ready for the day and for bed, and indulging in his multiple preferred methods of entertainment (i.e. games, toys, movies). See where I'm going here? Rest was impossible. Moreover, while I was committed to having a chill, low maintenance day, my attempt at rest had not resolved any of my critical pain levels. In fact, my shoulders, wrists and fingers were starting to hurt now as well.

My son had been in Pre-K part-time and I had never been more eager to drop him off than I was the following Monday morning. After dragging my feet along to get him into the school, I drove straight to the Emergency Room to be seen. Now, for those who know me, KNOW that I'm not going to the doctor, to Urgent Care, and the ER is the absolute last place on earth you will find me. I just believe in exhausting all my options at home first before going to see a doctor. Of course, if it's an emergency, that's a different story. And clearly, as a result of me checking in at the ER, I had an emergency. After registering and receiving a room, the NP on-call came in to discuss my symptoms. I explained to her what I was experiencing and she advised they run "what tests they could at the ER" just to get a baseline of what was going on. The tests were very limited, but she said there was inflammation in my body and that based on the symptoms I described combined with the test results, I should follow-up with my PCP and/or a Rheumatologist to rule out anything like lupus, rheumatoid arthritis, gout, or fibromyalgia. I wanted to skip the PCP and go straight to the Rheumatologist. I needed answers and I needed them now, so I wanted to see the specialist. The first rheumatologist's office I called advised I needed a referral from my PCP to be seen. So I called another. The second rheumatologist's office I called advised I needed a referral from my PCP. So I called another. And by the time I had called the third rheumatologist's office, I had gotten the picture. I needed a referral from my PCP.

Well, funny enough, at 32 years old, I didn't have a PCP. I had had one at some point, I'm sure, but had never had any health challenges or complications so I never felt like I needed to see a doctor regularly. Of course, I make sure my son sees his doctor regularly, but the only doctor I see is my OB-GYN, annually. Ironically, though, I had been telling my mom that I was getting older so I was going to book an appointment with a new PCP at the beginning of the year. I booked the appointment in January and the only availability they had was in May (the month we were in). I had received a phone call from the office the month prior, in April, cancelling my appointment because the doctor no longer worked for that practice and they were too short-staffed to take on any new patients. So, after calling multiple rheumatology offices with no success in scheduling an appointment, I called a family practice that the ER Nurse Practitioner recommended to establish new care with a PCP. The first available appointment wasn't until June 23rd. I had to wait about six weeks and though the NP prescribed me multiple steroids and medications for pain, I didn't have any intention of taking them. I wanted to know what was going on with me and how I could fix it, not mask whatever it was with pills.

The wait until my PCP visit was the longest six weeks of my life. Every night, I religiously spent hours on end researching my symptoms.

"Joint pain all over."

"Joint pain and muscle aches."

"Extreme fatigue."

"Chest pain and fatigue."

"Night sweats."

"Hair loss, chest pain, mouth ulcers, joint pain, muscle aches, extreme fatigue, face rash, extremely thirsty, headaches."

Every single search was returning the same results: Lupus.

I began flooding my mom and sister's messages with, "remember how I was telling you this a while ago…" or "you know how I be saying this…"

"Stay off the internet!" is what my mom would say. But eventually, I think she came to realize the dots were connecting as well. My symptoms were very real. And every day I was discovering a new one or one that I had been experiencing for a while and didn't know was correlated.

Sadly, researching my symptoms had become my new full-time job and crying was my part-time and I was putting in OT at both. I spent days in bed resting when I wasn't working, sometimes forcibly because I was in too much pain to do anything else. When I picked my son up from school, I pretended like I was just fine, played with him, helped him with homework, fed him, got him ready for bed, and boo-hoo cried after he went to sleep. Wake up, repeat.

Finally, the day arrived for me to see the PCP. I had never been so eager to go to the doctor's office in all my life. It wasn't the doctor I was eager to see. It was the answers that I needed. I wanted relief, physically and emotionally. Once again, I went down the list of my symptoms and the doctor told me she would run a series of tests to figure out what was going on. I left the office that Friday and I waited.

The following Tuesday I received an email from LabCorp with available test results. Of course, I didn't know what any of the results meant but I consulted with my very qualified best friend, Google. In short, my results pointed to what I already felt I knew. I even sent a few screenshots to my mom and she insisted I wait for the doctor's call before jumping to any conclusions. Within the hour, the doctor called:

"Ms. Brooks, we got your test results back and it indicates you have lupus and some other rheumatoid factor. I'm referring you to a rheumatologist because this is way out of my league."

That may have been a moment I was expected to cry, but honestly, I felt a sense of relief. For six weeks, I had endured an immense level of pain and other symptoms and I had to rely on Google for answers. It felt good to have my symptoms validated, to know that what I was feeling was real, that I wasn't crazy. I didn't want to claim lupus over my life, but I had also wanted to make peace with it if it had to become my reality. I didn't want the weight of devastation and grief to hit me as hard as the pain had for the past six weeks. On the flip side, it did also mean that I had a lifelong chronic illness. Out of nowhere. Just like that. It wasn't going away. It was here to stay.

The rheumatology referral felt like a golden ticket after waiting six weeks. What I hadn't taken into consideration, however, is how long I would have to wait to get an appointment to see a rheumatologist. The first office I called, which was about 10 minutes from my house, didn't have an appointment available for the next four months. So I called their partner office, which was 35 minutes from my house, and they had an appointment available two months out. Of course, two months meant another eight weeks of suffering, but it was better than 16, so I took it.

Those next eight weeks were excruciating. I experienced random face and lip rashes, hair loss, and more joint pain and muscle aches. My bed and I grew more and more acquainted as the fatigue consumed me. I was suffering, but I've never taken medication for anything. I didn't want to start popping pills, but every now and then, the pain was so unbearable that I gave in and took one, hoping for even the slightest bit of relief. It was becoming more and more evident that I was in the fight of my life - literally.

Finally, after waiting two months, I met with my new rheumatologist. My mom came along to the visit with me and we both agreed, the doctor didn't have the best bedside manners. You would think she was the one sitting in agonizing pain on a daily. But I digress. She reviewed my lab results sent over by my PCP and also instructed me to do more labs before leaving the visit. She also explained that my official diagnosis was Mixed Connective Tissue Disease (MCTD) and in short, it meant that I have an overlap between Systemic Lupus Erythematosus (SLE) and Rheumatoid Arthritis (RA). She explained that my lupus markers were very high and that she highly recommended medication as part of my treatment plan. She further explained that hydroxychloroquine was a lupus staple medication that protects one's organs from being impacted by lupus. It was considered a "low dose" lupus medication and then there was methotrexate, which was a stronger lupus medication. She didn't believe the hydroxychloroquine would help me much because my lupus markers were so significantly high. But I still settled for the low dose medicine and went on my way. I didn't want to go from taking no medication whatsoever to taking "high dose" meds daily. I figured I would start small and see if the "low dose" meds helped at all before advancing to stronger medication.

Rheumatoid Arthritis is an autoimmune disease that attacks your body's healthy tissues causing joint pain and inflammation in the body. Lupus is also an autoimmune disease that causes the immune system to attack its own healthy tissues. As a result, this also leads to inflammation in the body, which in turn, can lead to permanent tissue damage affecting vital organs like the heart, kidneys, liver, lungs and brain. These are unavoidable, incurable, lifelong chronic illnesses. Despite their debilitating physical effects, they have doubly forced me to fight - not only for my physical life, but also for my sanity.

It took me a month before I cracked open the bottle and began taking the pills daily. Transparently speaking, when I did, I felt defeated. I felt like I gave lupus the victory over my life. I felt like I claimed it in that moment. It became so real that I really had an illness and I now had to take medication daily in an effort to live. The worst part is, after three months, I had been taking the medicine every day to no avail. I was not getting any better. In fact, I felt worse. That's not to say the medicine made me worse, but that's just how little the medicine did for me. I had to remind myself that the doctor did say its primary use was for organ protection, but my joint pain was overtaking me. I explained that to my doctor at a follow-up visit. She looked at me as though she didn't believe me, but my lab work revealed that my lupus had, in fact, gotten worse. I sensed an "I told you so" moment when she recommended the "high dose" medication again. I accepted the prescription, because at that point, what choice did I have?

After three weeks of being on methotrexate, I felt as close to normal as I had in eight months. When I went for a rheumatology visit, I told my doctor, "I feel good!" She was excited to hear that, told me I didn't have to return for three months, and sent me for routine labs. The next day her office called and told me to stop taking the methotrexate. My lab results were in, and in just three weeks, the medication had significantly lowered my white blood cell count. I fought tooth and nail not to be on that medication, then I finally took it. And when I began to feel a sense of normalcy again, although because of meds, it was snatched right back from me within an instant. I was back to square one. Back to being in pain every day. I felt myself sinking into depression because this was not the quality of life I wanted to live. It was not what I deserved. I was frustrated. Overwhelmed. Discouraged. Angry. Infuriated.

I couldn't understand - why me? Why must I suffer this way? What have I done to deserve this? Why hasn't God shown up for me yet?

Why God?! Why haven't You shown up for ME yet?!

"My God, My God, why have You forsaken Me? Why are You so far from helping Me, And from the words of My groaning? O My God, I cry in the daytime, but You do not hear; And in the night season, and am not silent" (Psalm 22: 1-2, KJV).

I cried out to God in the morning, in the noontime and at night and He would not answer me. Wasn't I still His child? I felt forgotten. Disowned. Unloved. I was fighting for my life and I felt alone.

Then, one day, I decided to try Him one more time. With tears in my eyes and outstretched hands, I said, "God, I need You. I can't do this by myself. Could you show up for me? Could you do this for me, God? Please!"

Then I heard Him whisper back to me:

"I will never leave you nor forsake you."

"I will strengthen you; I will surely help you; I will uphold you with My righteous right hand."

"No weapon formed against you shall prosper."

"I will not put more on you than you can bear."

"I can do anything but fail."

I was reminded of His love for me. Briefly, I was convinced that my diagnoses were the Lord's doing. Once reality kicked in, I realized that this was the work of the devil. God is only of everything good and perfect. I also realized that I needed to move past my diagnoses. It's not going anywhere, but I still have plenty of places to go. I have a son to raise, goals to reach, people to help, a purpose to fulfill. So yes, I did throw a little pity party. But party's over! I'm reclaiming what's mine!

Every time I feel the need to wallow in despair, I tell myself to GET UP! It's easy to make excuses and I've never chosen the easy path. I've always earned what's mine. This victory will be no different!

Even when my wrists are aching and my fingers too, I GET UP every day and work on manuscripts. My purpose is making writers published authors. I owe it to myself and to those I serve to fulfill that purpose.

Even when the fatigue is so overwhelming and I just want to lay in my bed and rest, I still GET UP and show up for my family, my friends and my community.

Even with an aching body, I still GET UP and play with my son. I ensure he's well taken care of, he's healthy and he's happy every single day, despite how

I'm feeling. I still give him my best because that's what he deserves.

My purpose is greater than my pain. True enough, I'm not the same person I once was. In fact, I'm still grieving her. Getting Up looks differently than it did a year ago. However, to ensure that I'm able to GET UP as the new me while simultaneously taking care of myself, I implement a few personal principles in my life.

1. *No is a complete sentence.* This is difficult for people to understand when they're used to you being the "yes" girl. Know that it is well past time for you to start distributing some nos and don't feel guilty if you get a little generous with them.
2. *Rest is not optional, it's mandatory.* Having an autoimmune disease requires a great deal of rest and recovery, from even the simplest, smallest tasks. Be sure to develop a healthy rest and sleep regimen and do not deviate from it. Make it a priority because your body needs it.
3. *Pace yourself.* You don't have the same body you used to have, so you can't do everything on the same level. In some instances that require you to show up on the same level, like parenting for instance, learn to pace yourself by making adjustments where available. If I know my son and I are running around playing

outside or raking the yard, we're not running around or doing yard work the next day too. We'll have to find something a little less physically demanding, but equally engaging, to do. Or, if I know I have upcoming travel, I will cancel all plans days before and days after because I know I need to rest up to travel and I need to recover after.

4. *Grant yourself grace.* Battling chronic illness is not easy. It requires a great deal of unlearning and relearning your own self. As long as you're doing your best, know that that is always good enough!

5. *Avoid the naysayers*. Everyone is not going to understand your journey. They're not going to understand the magnitude of your pain when you communicate your symptoms. Some may even doubt you're telling the truth. Those people are not for you. Run from them and embrace those who show you real love and genuine concern and care.

A year ago, I could've never imagined this is where life would lead. But I'm here. Living with Lupus has been a complete nightmare. Every day, it seems I'm faced with new challenges, new symptoms, new fears. But God promised me LIFE, and LIFE more abundantly! Despite the chronic pain you may be enduring as a result of your diagnosis, let me encourage you to GET UP! You are still here for a reason. God's got a plan for you.

Whitney L. Brooks is a mom, serial entrepreneur and 6X published author. In 2015, Whitney transitioned to full-time business ownership as Co-Founder of **Patience for Patients, LLC**, a family-owned and operated non-medical homecare agency that provides quality personal care and companionship services to the geriatric population. As a multi-passionate entrepreneur who holds a BA in English with a minor in Creative Writing, she also began freelance editing for first-time authors and small business owners in 2016. Feeling a sense of obligation to fill the gap for first-time authors who had developed an immense level of trust in her, Whitney expanded her editing side hustle into a full-service publishing firm to provide guidance on the self-publishing process. Now, as CEO and Publisher of **Empower Her Publishing, LLC**, Whitney offers an all-inclusive, educational approach for women of influence to publish their experiences and expertise, thereby contributing to the growth of their brands and businesses. Additionally, after reaching and sustaining a significant level of success as a full-time business owner, Whitney birthed *The Millennial Mamapreneur* brand that helps highly ambitious moms develop the confidence and clarity to build six-figure brands while staying home with their babies. She provides foundational strategies to launch and grow successful businesses through her book, *Walk Into It: 7 Steps to Develop Confidence as an Emerging Entrepreneur*, online courses and consulting services. Moreover, Whitney is passionate about creating platforms for women entrepreneurs to shine and she does so through collaboration books, speaking engagements and her infamous Ultimate Girl Boss Pop-Up Experience events. Whitney is also the Founder of **Author Ave**, a social hub for new and aspiring authors to network and learn from their peers and industry experts, and the **Girl, Get Up Movement**, created to celebrate women living with autoimmune diseases, chronic illnesses and pain and to educate the community on the various impacts these health challenges have on their loved ones. She is also a proud member of Iota Phi Lambda Sorority, Incorporated. Whitney's greatest mission in life is to live life intentionally while hopefully impacting lives along the way. Whitney currently resides in Richmond, VA with her son, Malachi, and their family dog, Chance.

Connect with Whitney:
Linktr.ee/iamwhitneyb
Facebook: Whitney L. Brooks
Instagram: @themillennialmamapreneur

Schizophrenic Body
Trimika Cooper

Having an autoimmune disease can be physically and mentally challenging. It brings on a flood of emotions and unbearable pain. It's even harder when it's unpredictable. At the age of 19, I was diagnosed with Hypothyroidism which is a condition in which my thyroid gland doesn't produce enough thyroid hormone. I was always tired, and no matter how much I would cut back on eating, I would still gain weight. I also had migraines so bad that they caused nauseousness and blurry vision. I became depressed and at first, I figured it was from the weight gain. Then my muscles began to ache and I was weak all the time. I knew something else was wrong. I've never been a fan of taking medicine, not even for pain. After multiple blood tests, it was determined that I would have to take a daily thyroid hormone replacement because I have Thyroid Disease. One pill a day, I could deal with that. But then I was also required to take a shot once a month and a pill twice a day for the migraines. Additionally, I have to get my labs checked every three months and it seems like every time my results come back, my medicine dose has to be increased or decreased. This is not encouraging at all. I hate taking medicine as it is and my thyroid levels are never where they should be.

As years have passed, I've had children and I now have three grandchildren. I'm getting older and I realize our bodies change with age, but my body feels extremely different; it has for some time now. In December 2020, during Covid, things began to change for the worse and rapidly. I woke up one morning and tried to turn over in bed and I know for a fact my body said, "Where do you think you're going?" I tried to laugh it off and attempted to Get Up again and the pain that came from my joints was unbearable. My physique said, "I repeat, where do you think you're going?" That is the moment I realized either I was going crazy or my body was actually talking to me. Did my body just ask me a question? I now believe I have schizophrenia of the body. I had a cold and some muscle aches but this pain right here was different. When I tell you I could not get out of the bed… I felt defeated trying. As I lay in awe of this episode, I began to pray. After I prayed, I called my PCP, Dr. Sang's, office. I explained to the nurse the events of my morning and she told me I might have the flu which causes muscle aches. Now I have had the flu before and this wasn't it. This was non-identical and not related to flu. Nevertheless, I scheduled an appointment to see Dr. Sang. Of course, the earliest date available was two weeks out.

One week before my appointment I started having pain in my right ankle. It began to bruise, swell, and throb like a toothache. I bought some compression socks to see if that would make a difference, but to no avail, the pain increased. Something is definitely wrong, I thought to myself.

"Dr. Sang, I'm telling you there's something going on with my body. I can't put my finger on it but I feel different. I take my thyroid medicine every morning on an empty stomach, but still feel fatigued, even after going to bed early. You keep putting me on these steroids for joint pain, which isn't helping with any of the pain but causing me to gain more weight. And I still haven't received any answers as to why I'm in so much pain. Look at my ankle, it's so swollen that it's bruised from the stretching. At times I feel as if my anatomy doesn't like itself. I awake to parts of my hull unfamiliar with its counterparts. You can say my body parts are arguing with each other, if that makes sense to you. Even though our internal body parts don't have the ability to communicate the way we do, our nervous system does use electrical and chemical means to help all parts of the body to transmit with each other. I know I sound crazy but I feel really off on the inside and I don't like this feeling. Maybe it's something mental, I'm not sure, but something has to change and I need answers. Especially after the way my body hurt the other week as I was trying to Get Up out of bed. My body literally laughed at me. That was not normal pain and not symptoms of the flu."

"Trimika, I understand your concerns. And no, I don't think it's mental, but I can do some extensive testing and blood work to figure out what's going on. Let's work together on finding a solution for all of this. Once the test results come back, I will call you in to go over everything. In the meantime, I want to put you on a steroid pack to see if it helps with that ankle swelling."

"Now here we go again. More medicine. And steroids at that."

"I know Trimika, but we have to relieve some of the swelling in that ankle. Now follow the instructions on the package. The first day you will take six, the next day take five, and each day go down with the dosage. Let's see if that will help."

"Thanks, Dr. Sang."

As days go by, my body continues to hurt, especially my knee and ankle. Of course, the steroids didn't help with any swelling. Lord, what is going on with my body? I'm leaning and depending on you, Jesus. This pain causes you not to want to go anywhere or do anything. It takes a lot out of a person when you're in constant pain. This can cause a damper on relationships, especially when people don't realize the magnitude of pain you're experiencing. Being an independent person who is not used to asking for help makes you feel weak. So you endure the pain as much as you can in silence.

A week later, I got a call from Dr. Sang to come into the office. As I sat and listened to her go over my test results, she explained that my tests show that I have lupus. She goes on to say that about six percent of people with lupus have underactive thyroid, or hypothyroidism. It was a lot to take in and I couldn't help but cry out, "Lord, by your stripes, I am healed." Of course, I knew nothing about lupus so this was a sticker shock to me. Dr. Sang gave me a referral to see a Rheumatoid Specialist. All the information was like a foreign language to me and too much to inhale. I left Dr. Sang's office limping because my ankle was still swollen. I was overwhelmed with emotions and felt bewildered.

Hearing the news that I have lupus did not help me at all. I was still in the dark as to what it really meant. What am I supposed to do? Is it curable? How long does it last? Is it permanent? Question after question consumed my thoughts. Since I was unsure about what it meant, I decided to wait to tell my family until after I saw the specialist. I don't have health insurance; therefore, I had to pay out of pocket. Yet another blow that consumed my thoughts. Once I got the call for the specialist appointment, the earliest they could see me was four months out. FOUR MONTHS! I asked to be put on the cancellation list just in case I could be seen earlier. The specialist did send me an order to get lab work done as well as x-rays of my knees so she could have some answers for me during my visit. I thought that was good because by this point, my ankle and knee were so swollen. I couldn't wear a shoe and could barely bend my knee.

James 5:14: Is anyone among you sick? Let them call the elders of the church to pray over them and anoint them with oil in the name of Jesus.

Unfortunately, because of Covid, church was only being held online. So I got in my prayer closet with my anointing oil and I prayed and anointed myself. I asked God to heal me. I know my time is not His time, but I knew in due time He would heal me. As I waited for my appointment, I did a lot of Google searches. Google will scare the mess out of you but it also opened my eyes to things that I had been dealing with that I had no idea were as a result of having lupus.

Throughout the years, anytime I was out in the sun, my body would ache or my face would swell, especially around my eyes. My skin would burn even while using sunscreen and I'd always have a rash on my face in a butterfly shape under my eyes and down my nose. This information really brought more awareness to things I had been enduring throughout the years. I think my body does have schizophrenia.

Finally, the day arrived for me to see the Rheumatoid Specialist and my ankle and knee were still very swollen. It looked as if I had elephantiasis. I had been out of work for the last four days because I could barely walk and my joints hurt so bad. I really needed some answers from the rheumatologist. When Dr. Floyd entered the room, she greeted me and immediately noticed the swelling in my leg and ankle. She asked how long it had been swollen and I told her about six months. I told her it took four months for me to get an appointment with her. Dr. Floyd went over my lab results and explained that I have Systemic Lupus Erythematosus (SLE), which is an autoimmune disease where the body's defense system mistakenly attacks healthy cells and tissues, causing damage to many parts of the body. She confirmed that I also have Lupus Dermatitis, and Rheumatoid Arthritis. Dr. Floyd explained the pain in my knee was the result of a pillar cyst in my knee cap. Every time I would bend it, puss seeped out and drained down into my ankle. Wow, for months I had endured so much pain to find out it's a cyst in my knee.

That visit was a hard one but I was glad I had some answers. Dr. Floyd recommended that I change my eating, cut back on my sugar intake, eat more fruits and vegetables and of course, prescribed more medication. Another steroid along with two different types of Lupus medicines as well as pain medicine, all twice a day. Not to mention, my thyroid medicine and two migraine suppressants. That's a total of seven pills twice a day. An abundance of medicine in which I did not want to take, but I knew I had to. I also got a cortisone shot in my knee. All this in one day was a flood of emotions. The more I endure, the more I've come to realize that I have schizophrenia of the body.

To say the least, I have been taking all this medication and still feel as if nothing is working or I'm having so many side effects. Of course, the doctor takes you off one medicine just to put you on another. I am beginning to feel like a lab rat and I feel like enough is enough.

Having lupus can be very unpredictable. One day you feel fine, the next day you're struggling to Get Up. My family has had to really step in to help me out more, especially with household chores. The rheumatoid arthritis in my hands has become quite a burden for me. I can barely make a fist or even pick up a plate. The tips of my fingers are beginning to curve and my knuckles swell to the point they look deformed. To say the least, the pain is insufferable. Having lupus has been a psychological roller coaster. I love my job but there are some days I can't make it because of the pain in my joints. I have noticed that stress or being overworked brings on a flare up. I have to wear leg warmers in the winter time to help filter out the cold air on my knees. I've definitely learned that lupus + cold weather = major flare ups. I also have to stay out of direct sunlight. Waking up in the mornings with my face swollen where I can't see my eyes has become my normal. I had to realize my normal is definitely different from other people's normal and I'm ok as long as I can bear the pain.

My doctor recommended that I get the Covid shots. Everyone who got it before me said that the second shot was worse than the first. Well my experience was very different. I got the Moderna Covid vaccine and I thought it was going to take me out. I had to go to the hospital because I was so dehydrated and weak because I couldn't keep anything down. I received IV fluids for hours and I was so puny I couldn't hold my head up. The doctor said that my body thought the shot was an invasion and started to fight it. That's the schizophrenia part of my body. Even though I take my medicine, I never know when it will resurface or how long it will last.

Having an autoimmune disease that you have no control over or not even sure of all the triggers can be vexing, but I have to continue to Get Up and be a wife, Get Up and be a mother, Get Up and go to work. Modifying my lifestyle has been vigorous, but a must in order for me to see results in how my schizophrenic body reacts. After having a seizure a couple of months ago, the doctors couldn't tell me why so I decided to stop taking my medicine and cut out all meat, except turkey. This includes processed meat. I also began to juice my fruits and vegetables. I have lost some weight, but the inflammation in my body hasn't changed. My joint pain has definitely increased where some days I can barely walk and the rheumatoid arthritis in my hands have gotten worse. I'm hoping that it's just my body trying to adjust to no medicine and no meat.

Lupus flare ups have disallowed me to do certain things that I had planned. I had a book launch in Houston, Texas and I couldn't attend because of a flare up. It's to the point I don't like planning things because I'm scared I will have to cancel. This can be very disheartening as well as depressing. It makes you feel like your independence is being taken away especially when your regular activities are challenging to do because of your pain. It's one thing to realize that on a normal day you will have pain but it's the unexpected pains that shock you. I've learned that having a good support system helps a lot. Being open and honest with yourself, your family, and your job about the things you're able to do is important. I will continue to lean and depend on Jesus through it all. Jeremiah 30:17 says, "For I will restore health unto thee, and I will heal thee of thy wounds, saith the Lord." I will definitely stand on His word. I hope my story can help someone who may be going through the same or a similar autoimmune disease. Keep your head up and trust God.

Trimika Cooper is from Chadbourn, NC, but is a resident of Charlotte, NC where she lives with her husband, Genatus Cooper. She is the mother of four children: Sharmane, Destinee', Marcus and Jayden; grandmother to three granddaughters: Amina, Angel, and Anissa, and also has a fur baby named Grace. She is an ordained minister who loves helping those in need. Trimika is CEO of Cooper's Creative Stylez Balloon Decor, Faith, Family, and Fabulous Hair T-shirt line, Visionary Author of Amazon's #1 Best-Selling book, *4Ms:*

Muted Molestation that Manifested Mentally, Co-Author of Amazon's #1 Best-Selling book, *Reclaiming My Life*, which has a podcast on Youtube, also airs on SMENLIGHTMENT MEDIA, WESL Radio, Rejoice 93.7, and PRAISE BY GRACE RADIO in all 50 states and over 125 countries, Co-Author of Amazon's #1 Best-Selling book, *Resisting Temptation: Overcoming and Surviving Addiction*, as well as Co-Author of Amazon's Best-Selling book, *The Final Chapter: Reclaiming My Life After the Storm*. Trimika also works a full-time job as an Assistant Director at Harris Learning Academy.

Keep in touch with Trimika:
Facebook: Min Trimika Cooper
Facebook: Coopers Creative Stylez
Instagram: Coopers_Creative_Stlyez
TikTok: @Cooperscreativestylez

The Battle is Not Over
Claudia Massey

"God is our refuge and strength, a very present help in trouble" (Psalm 46:1).

I was only 18 years old when I first experienced the most excruciating pain of my life. It was a constant stabbing sensation in my right arm and both my wrists. I had never felt this level of pain before so I was extremely concerned. I was a cable winder for Escod Industries in Clarkton, NC and thought that was contributing to the pain in my arms. The doctor told my mom I had tendinitis, gave me a brace and sent me on my way. I continued going to work, never missing a day, just as I had never missed a day of school from Kindergarten through 12th grade. In addition to the pain, I was extremely fatigued. I had been experiencing fatigue consistently for at least three years. As a teen living in the country, I worked in the tobacco fields. I came home one day overly exhausted. Since I didn't like being outside, my mom thought I was trying to get out of going to work and shut down my hopes of taking a day off before I could even attempt to ask. Truthfully, though, the heat was wearing me down.

In 1991, I was 19 years old and pregnant with my first child. I was about seven months into the pregnancy, and again, was in excruciating pain. I couldn't stand to walk or to do anything really. My entire body cried out for help. My doctor at the time told me I was constipated. To me, that just didn't sound right. I was experiencing an indescribable and most undesirable pain one could imagine. It literally had me bed bound for days. Then, one night about two years later, when I was nine months pregnant with my second child, I thought I was going to die. My family and I went out to Dale's Seafood and I'll never forget, I had hamburger steak and went home happy and full. Later in the night, here we go again - I was in agonizing pain. I felt like I couldn't breathe. It didn't feel like labor; it was 100 times worse. My husband at the time drove me to the hospital and out of all times, it seemed like he just wasn't driving fast enough. I was crying, screaming and yelling, "DRIVE THIS CAR!" I arrived at the hospital and don't remember too much because the pain wouldn't allow me to be alert. That night, I birthed my beautiful baby girl and the doctor (my doctor wasn't on call), who was one I hadn't seen before, walked over and asked me if I had sickle cell. I told her no. She tested me anyway - my baby as well - and told me, "Mrs. Brooks (at that time), you have sickle cell disease. You and your baby almost didn't survive."

After years of knowingly living with the disease now, I understand that the reason why we almost didn't survive is because when you are in a sickle cell crisis, the blood isn't flowing normally. Instead, the blood becomes crescent-shaped and stuck which causes pain. Subsequently, if the blood isn't flowing, it cuts off oxygen to vital organs. Though labor and delivery was over, I was still in a crisis. So much pain. I was trying to process it all. Thank God my baby was ok and she tested negative for sickle cell. I wasn't knowledgeable about sickle cell then, but I now know with me having sickle cell that if her dad had also had it, or even the sickle cell trait, that my baby would have had sickle cell disease too.

Instances like mine are reasons why it's important for us to really educate ourselves on autoimmune diseases and how they can affect us and our loved ones. After learning about sickle cell disease and its genetic impact, I had my oldest daughter tested and thankfully, she only has the sickle cell trait. As my daughters got older, I then taught them the importance of having sickle smart conversations with potential mates before considering beginning a family. Labor is a breeze compared to a sickle cell crisis. I would endure it for a week over a sickle cell crisis for an hour. After delivering my second child, I was in a pain crisis for two weeks. I could barely walk, hold my baby, or anything. I would lay in bed and cry so much begging God to take the pain away. I promised Him if He healed me that just as soon as I could walk, I would walk to the altar and give my life to Him. The next Saturday I was able to attend church and I was so grateful that I ran to the altar.

There's one thing about a sickle cell crisis, and that is, most times they come without warning. After my second child, I knew I didn't want any more children because pregnancy was a huge flare for me. Well, God had other plans for my life because my birth control failed me and here I was expecting again. Ohhhh my goodness, did I suffer. This pregnancy with my last baby had me in some kind of pain. I remember the night I was in crisis at nine months pregnant AGAIN. I suffered that entire night because I wanted to see my kids off to school the next morning and didn't want them to know I was going to the hospital so they wouldn't worry about me. Just as soon as they got on the bus, I left for the hospital. I don't remember getting there or being transported to a high risk hospital. Yes, I arrived at one hospital and they transported me to another and I have no recollection of it. Sickle cell pain is the kind of pain that makes you cry out, "CUT MY ARM OFF!" You will ask somebody, anybody, to cut whatever off that is hurting and ACTUALLY MEAN IT!!!

Before becoming pregnant again with my last child, I had promised my grandmother who later passed, that if I ever had another baby (because I didn't think I would), that I would breastfeed. So even in my pain, I kept my promise and nursed my baby that it hurt me to even hold. Well, I started something because seven months postpartum, I was bicycling and the strain and stress on my legs from doing so caused me to go into a crisis. My baby was so spoiled that she wouldn't let anyone hold her. My mom tried her best with her but couldn't stop her from crying. Eventually, she had to bring her to the hospital, put her in my arms and let me nurse her while I was suffering! A mother's love is unfailing!

That wasn't the only time I sacrificed my pain for my child. She was about seven years old and got sick and had to stay in the hospital overnight. I was in crisis but wouldn't tell anyone. I didn't want to leave my baby so I asked the nurse if they could see me in the room with her. Of course, she told me I had to be seen in the Emergency Room, so I refused treatment. Again, I suffered and silently cried all night. When I say I will lay MY life on the line for my children, believe it. My daughter went to school the next day. I called my mom and told her I needed to desperately go to the doctor. She picked me up and as soon as my doctor saw me he said "go to the hospital." I went there to find out I had to have my gallbladder removed. Ironically, I had just been by my sister's side, who had sickle cell anemia, five months prior as she had her gallbladder removed. Sadly, my sister passed away from sickle cell complications in 2010. She was only 26 years old. Gallbladder issues, more specifically gallstones, are common among sickle cell patients. This happens when too many sickle cells burst and release their contents into the bloodstream.

Although painful, the gallstones have not been the most horrific part of my health journey. I take the punches and roll with them but sometimes, the devil likes to creep in and try to steal my joy. There have been times during travels, like when my husband and I went out of town and were having the most amazing evening. We came in from dinner and before I knew it, I was saying, "get me to a hospital ASAP!" I could say it's embarrassing for EMT to come to your hotel room and take you to the hospital, but I barely remember. I can laugh about it because God is so good to me. I don't sit around and feel sorry for myself. When I'm in pain, I fight! I think of my children and my goals and I know I owe it to them to continue the fight.

There are other instances, however, when I'm not able to physically "Get Up!" One morning in September of 2019, I had a headache that was so intense that I couldn't see straight, couldn't hold my head up, and couldn't make it out of the bed to perform my daily tasks. I literally slept for hours on end. I couldn't do anything else. When I finally got up, the right side of my face felt a little numb. I knew then that I really needed to go to the hospital, but I didn't want to go. What led to me going was listening to my daughter tell me I was acting like my late mother who had refused to go to the hospital. That really clicked for me, and as bad as the struggle was to get dressed and make it out the door, I went. Once I arrived, the medical staff performed test after test after test. They concluded I suffered a TIA, or mini stroke.

Ultimately, the medical team at MCV Hospital felt like the TIA was a result of me having sickle cell disease. As a result, I had to start monthly blood transfusions. The goal of the exchange blood transfusions was to remove the "bad blood" and infuse "good blood" into me. Over the course of the three years that I received the transfusions, I sometimes had reactions to them that would cause me to urinate blood. Eventually, that's why they ended. Truthfully, I'm not even sure if the transfusions were necessary. They were recommended to prevent clotting (that sickle cell causes); but the reality is, like one sickle cell doctor in clinic pointed out: When sickle cell patients who are kids have strokes - like my sister who had sickle cell anemia and had a stroke at age 11 - it's a given that it's sickle cell related. When sickle cell adults have strokes, however, it's not always as a result of sickle cell, because many adults who do not have sickle cell also have strokes. Nevertheless, it was a part of my journey. It's an unknown I'll never know. A hard unknown, to say the least. The transfusions were overwhelming, but I am unstoppable.

When you experience a sickle cell crisis, there is no worse pain in this world so inevitably, it made me strong. If I can conquer that, when I'm weak, cut up from port surgery, cut up from a heart implant, experiencing low blood pressure, always feeling tired from being anemic, I REFUSE to lay down when I'm not crippled as I've been. I tell myself, "Girl, Get Up! You can move, so move! You can cook, so cook! You can travel so travel!" My disease does not control me, my mind does! I also have osteoarthritis in my knees. My knee has been so swollen to the point I couldn't squat to sit on the toilet. It was in so much pain. The first time it flared up really bad, I was in New Orleans. It happened on the plane traveling there. I didn't allow it to keep me in my room, however. I went to celebrate my friend's birthday and although I was walking VERY slowly, I was still walking.

In addition to sickle cell, I also have uveitis, which is an eye condition. I've had to have countless injections, several eye surgeries and even lost sight for two days in my right eye. As a matter of fact, I was out of town to shoot a movie and lost my sight a day before shooting. Guess what? I filmed the movie blind and never told anyone until the movie came out.

This has been a battle for 12 years but because I "get up," I'm winning! People often ask how I do all that I do with my illnesses. I tell them because I'm still alive. My sister died at age 26 from sickle cell. My mother passed away from a stroke and a heart attack. I might be in pain, might be labeled; I might even be weak some days, but EVERY DAY that God gives me breath and my limbs can move, I GET UP!! To all of the ladies who are battling an illness, keep fighting! And on your good days, don't allow the enemy to control your mind. GIRL, GET UP!!

As you may realize, even my doctor wasn't sickle cell educated. Unfortunately, back in the 60's and 70's, it wasn't talked about enough. People were just making babies. Today, there are a lot of resources and information to educate you on sickle cell. WE can stop bringing babies into the world to suffer and die. I urge everyone to be tested and to be sickle smart!

In loving memory of my sister, Sickle Cell Warrior, Quinica Smith.

Claudia R. Massey is a resident of Richmond, Virginia where she devotes much of her time being a wife to her husband, James, and together, they have eight children, three of whom they adopted out of foster care. She is the Co-Founder of Patience for Patients, LLC, a non-medical homecare agency that provides personal care and companionship services to the geriatric population. Claudia attends Courthouse Road Church of Seventh-Day Adventists where she is a devoted member and Women's Ministry Leader. She is a Radio Host at Rejoice WBTK 1380 AM, a TV Host at Preach The Word Worldwide Network, a Certified Life and Wellness Coach, a 6X best-selling author, and a Columnist for Diva Dynasty Magazine. Claudia is also a Podcast Host of Reclaiming My Life on Rejoice 93.7 FM, WESL 1490, Praise By Grace radion station, SM Enlightenment Radio, and Ruff Boyz Radio. Claudia's most recent achievement is being an Honoree for The President Biden Volunteer Award!

In her very spare time, she enjoys traveling with her family, feeding the homeless at local shelters and giving back to those in need through a family initiative she founded in memory of her mom, Rena's New Life Ministry. On August 2, 2018, Rena's New Life Ministry was established as a community service organization to give back to those in need, much like Rena did. Moreover, Claudia spearheaded adoption of an Adventist Church School in North Carolina where her daughters attended and her mother once taught and she provides a yearly scholarship in her mother's name along with a monthly college incentive. Each year on August 2nd in commemoration of her mother's transition, Claudia decided to turn her negative emotions into positive energy by starting a back-to-school initiative with school supplies and resources for underprivileged inner city youth. Rena's New Life Ministry also offers a multi-state Secret Santa Christmas Miracle Shopping Experience for Struggling Single Parents and much more. These efforts of giving are truly from the heart, with the goal of being a blessing to others as they prepare to establish "new life" among their hardships. Additionally, Claudia sought to keep the memory and legacy of Rena alive, through this ministry as a symbol of her "new life" here on earth.

To those who know Claudia, she is known as one of the sweetest and strongest people one will ever meet. Her compassion for people, even during her own adversities and trials with sickle cell is truly unmatched.

Keep in touch with Claudia:
Facebook: @coachclaudiamassey
Instagram: @coachclaudiamassey
Website: contactclaudiamassey.com

Thank You to My Pre-Order Supporters!

Patricia Finney

Trinity Creations LLC

Facebook: Patricia Finney

Instagram: @Pfinney0316

Tat Chancy

ThissandThat

ThissandThat.com

Facebook: @tatchancy

Instagram: @whatchawant

Joanne Johnson

Joanne Johnson Tax Services

LinkedIn: linkedin.com/in/joanne-t-johnson-7663b613/

Melissa Mckoy

Shena's Place Uniforms and Boutique 0

Facebook: Melissa McKoy

Teneshia Phillips

TP Management Group

www.tpmgmtgroup.com

Facebook: @tpmgmtgroup

Instagram: @tpmgmtgroup

Josephine Sagini

Humanecare Residential Homes

humanecareresidentialhomes.com

Angel Burney

Reclaiming My Life: angelburney.com, Shower Down (music single): angelburney.hearnow.com

Facebook: Angel Autry Burney; Faith Assembly Outreach Center

Instagram: @AngelBurney

Tonya White

Tonya's Tax Prep & More

Facebook: @Tonya'sTaxPrep&More

Instagram: @tonyastaxprep

Ursula Jones

Prissy Tx Notary

Prissytxnotary.com

Facebook: @Ursula Priscilla Jones

Instagram: @prissyjvlogs

Regina McIntyre

Songwriter

Metamorphosis
Lare Ngofa

On the inside of my college class ring, the word 'Metamorphosis" is inscribed. I remember thinking about how to make it feel special and create a memory with it, and the word just came to me. For me, my undergraduate experience was a complete transformation. There was personal growth, mental, physical, and emotional struggles, and most importantly, there was triumph in the face of darkness. Less than 10 years removed from that, I see not only much more growth, but I also see how the decisions that were made by the emerging adult version of myself laid the foundation for me to create the life that I had dreamed for myself, however unattainable I thought it would be. I am not quite sure where the phrase "comparison is the thief of joy" comes from, but it most certainly has been the case for me. It has not only robbed me of life, joy, and peace, but also of healing.

I remember times during middle school years that I'd wake up with pain so strong, it would sometimes take the breath out of me. During those years, I was told I was too young to be tired, too young to have any serious kinds of issues, and so I spent a large part of my younger years telling myself that I was just catastrophizing and that what I was feeling was just in my head. Fast forward about five years later, after intense bouts of painful attacks, I was unable to deny that there was something majorly happening with my health, and at 17 years old, I was filled with equal parts trepidation as I was with fear.

The first time I'd heard the words premenstrual dysphoric disorder (PMDD), I was reading a random magazine and just happened to stumble across the symptoms listed at the time. They sounded a little too familiar: irritability, trouble concentrating, sleep issues, and severe uterine cramping. I brought it up to my OB-GYN the following year and she had actually said that she was going to mention it to me at that appointment. That, combined with my already established migraine diagnosis from the previous year, felt comforting to have labels to describe what was happening in my body. However, it was also terrifying as I was now faced with having two chronic health issues and the accompanying prescription medications for them by the time I turned 18.

As an evolving adult, I heard countless times how I was not invincible and had many older family members encouraging me to be mindful that the decisions that I'd make today would affect my life years ahead. What was more interesting to me at that point in my life was that I'd already been thinking about that. The thoughts had ravaged my mind multiple times over the last year and a half of my secondary education. Thoughts of whether or not I'd be able to have children, concern over my mental health ebbing and flowing, worries about how I would be able to manage a life in healthcare if I was struggling to manage my own pain in high school. There were so many thoughts that constantly told me that I was not strong enough, I did not have what it took, and that I would just be doomed to fail. With stress being my largest trigger for both my migraines and PMDD, I could not imagine a path forward that did not include my mostly living pain free and living the life I wanted to live - personally and professionally. How would I be able to travel? What if I had a migraine attack and I was not in a country with easy access to a neurologist? Would I be able to seriously consider medical school? Will I have to take medication for the rest of my life? If this pain I'm feeling now stays the same or even increases, what quality of life would I have?

I cannot tell you when I stopped having those specific thoughts, but what I can tell you is that my wakeup call was while sitting in my dorm room with my best friend and sister who told me that with all the stress, worry, and anxiety that I was going to die before I turned 30. I can hardly remember the conversation in totality, but that statement is forever burned into my memory. Anyone who suffers from chronic pain will tell you that the toll on your mental health is undeniable. There are days when my body cannot accomplish what my brain is telling me I need to do. There are days when both my brain and my body just cannot seem to get in sync with each other, and she was the first person (and likely the only person at that time) who was able to give me the jolt that I needed. I needed to hear those words, as sharp as she said them, because as someone who had dealt with suicidal ideations in their younger years, I very much knew I wanted to stick around a little longer. I knew that I had not accomplished what I was put here to do. I knew that there was still work for me to do. From that day, until now, any decision I have made for my life has been based on what I wanted to do and how it suits me. Not long after that conversation, I officially decided that I was rerouting and medical school was not going to be a part of my journey - at least for the time being. I transferred to the college of my choice and changed my major not long after. Those three decisions in hindsight are very minor, but for me, they were the start of me taking a stand for what was best in my life - without being encumbered by the opinions of others or the expectations of my parents. For me, the expectations placed on my shoulders weighed heavily, being my mother's oldest child and being first-generation American. Moreover, as the older sibling to two autistic boys, now men, it was of great importance to me to be financially situated by the time I was in my 30s to be able to secure a place for the three of us, in addition to the family I'd go on to create. The stress of trying to accommodate the outside world in my life, and trying to simultaneously live the life I wanted to live, while also managing chronic pain was clearly not working, and so I had to adapt.

That's not to say that things were easy. There was a layer of imposter syndrome as I had a friend in college who was recently diagnosed with endometriosis and there were two other friends I know who dealt with nerve pain. "I had more good days than they did so things can't be too bad for me then. I just need to adjust how I think about a few things and I'll be fine," was my thought. Until, my medication stopped working and I was again forced to deal with all of that pain in its full force. There were many tears shed in my dorm room, silently, not wanting to awake or alarm anyone because there wasn't anything they could do. I ended up having a flare with my PMDD on a weekend trip to visit my family and laid in a bathtub filled with scalding hot water crying out to God because I had run out of options. I hadn't felt heard in the moment, but things began to level out once again and I had more thoughts about my future and what it looked like. Age aside, I knew that God had not called me to a life of suffering, and so in the same way that I had researched PMDD after coming across it by chance, I began to research more natural ways to manage it as well as my migraines. I opened up to my close friends who were well aware of my medications and the importance of them in my daily life and I said by the time I turned 25, I would be off of them. It was a lofty goal, considering at that time I was taking four pills daily plus two more as needed for pain, but I also knew in my competitive spirit, I needed to give myself a challenge.

I began taking back pieces of my life bit by bit, becoming more involved in activities on campus. There were some hard days, but I quickly learned to be open and upfront with them so that I did not allow myself to suffer silently. There were times I would realize that I was closer to my menstrual cycle and knew that I could potentially have a flare up with my PMDD and I would take that time to get ahead with as much as I could. I prayed more, I meditated more, I took advantage of the down times that would be afforded to me by having my own apartment. I took every aspect of my life that I could control and made it fit within the confines of what seemed reasonable as someone dealing with chronic pain. I stopped limiting myself by others' beliefs and started to push myself to stand in my own truth, whatever that meant. When my PMDD or my migraines flared up, I unapologetically took the time I needed to rest and recover. I allowed myself to be supported more by the village I created for myself.

By the time I transferred to my alma mater, I wasn't near as many flares with my pain as I had before, and I feel very proud to say that I met my goal of being completely free of all my prescription medications by the time I was 25. There were a few hiccups along the way, but the journey was mine and I owned every part of it. I felt like I had finally gotten to a point where I didn't need to be fearful or worried about what the future may hold for me.

November 2020 would be the start of a new phase in my chronic pain journey, where I would spend four and a half months in a severe migraine crisis. I remember one day in the midst of that time thinking it was nowhere near this bad when I was 17 and 18. This was literally my worst nightmare. My partner would have to help me get into the bathtub to bathe, because I couldn't stand in the shower due to vertigo. Making myself one meal to eat would completely zap my energy for the rest of the day, struggling to have the energy to do the simplest tasks. Nothing was helping and I slowly came around to the idea that I would need to go back on prescription medications in order to see any real change in my pain levels. To say I was devastated would be an understatement. All of the work I had put in, all of the years I had spent learning my cycles, learning what my early migraine tells were, and I felt as if it had all been for naught.

Here I was, months away from 30 years old and feeling like I'm battling my body again for my life. The doubt started to creep in as it had done a decade before. I was making it more than it was. There were plenty of other people who had it worse than me and the difference was I had a little more life experience on my side to stop those thoughts in their tracks. Towards the end of my second month during this migraine attack, I made the decision that I was going to speak with my doctor about resuming some pharmaceutical support. I had no idea what I wanted to try but I was willing to throw everything I had at it. Because I already know the standard procedures, I knew that it would be wise to take a pregnancy test prior so that I would not have to worry about that going into my doctor's office. As my partner and I had been planning to conceive, it felt like a smart and preemptive decision, even though I had very little thoughts that I'd be pregnant because of the amount of pain that I'd been in preventing me from coming close to any level of cute. Days before Christmas, I took the pregnancy test and it came back negative - great, all clear for medication and I was hopeful that I'd be feeling some relief soon. I set up appointments with both my primary care doctor and neurologist, and as luck would have it, I had a positive pregnancy test at my primary care doctor's office. To their surprise I'm sure, I sat there in my sunglasses stunned, half confused and half irritated. That likely meant I was not going to be cleared for medication as I had hoped.

For three weeks, I wrestled with God ahead of my OB-GYN appointment. I knew I'd always desired to have children, but this was NOT how it was supposed to go. How can I force the child to go through all of the pain I'm dealing with? Was I actually pregnant? How would I manage to go through an entire 40 weeks of pregnancy with this level of pain? All the fears and anxieties had settled in within hours of me getting home from the doctor's office. I sat through and completed my work calls for the day and went through my usual routine that day. Then the next day I was hit with another wave of vertigo that kept me in bed for most of the day. With tears in my eyes, I was struggling to try and pray and the only thing that came into my mind was my life verse: Matthew 11:29-30, "Take my yoke upon you, and learn of me, for I am gentle and humble in heat, and you will find rest for your souls. For my yoke is easy and my burden is light." I just kept repeating it as much as I could and eventually I fell asleep. When I woke up, I felt so refreshed and rejuvenated that I ended up cooking a full meal that evening. I almost felt like I was back to normal, even though I was still in pain.

That one good day was all I needed to give me a little glimmer of hope. The second week after that doctor's appointment I realized that I hadn't had any missed menstrual periods and that I would be expecting it the week of my scheduled OB-GYN appointment. That gave the timeline I was on an entirely different perspective. While things were still very tentative, I felt like it made more sense to do what I could to shake this migraine and more importantly, get a blood test to confirm if I was pregnant. During that second week also came another day clouded by pain and lack of sleep. By this point, I was almost exclusively living in dark rooms and hushed voices. Early in the evening I just cried out to God, "I cannot do this without help. If you are calling me to do something, just tell me what it is. Am I supposed to rest? Am I to fight? Is there something I need to do? Just tell me so I can put this aside?" In that moment, I realized that I was speaking more to my current situation and not to my future. That felt like the difference between overcoming versus being overcome. It was very easy to continue to wallow in my cycle of pain, fatigue, and fear of the possibility of carrying a child with me through this, until that moment when I realized, no.

NO! I WOULD NOT accept that this is what this experience was going to be. I WOULD NOT allow the fears that I'd held for most of my life to this point come to fruition. If I had a choice in this, I was choosing to not stay in this space. I knew it was important that I speak to my future and what I saw in it. I saw myself living pain free. I saw myself back to resting when I needed to rest to take care of my body. I saw myself welcoming my first born into my heart and into my life with a fierce and extraordinary love. And from that moment on, I decided to get up every day and take small steps towards recovery. The night before I went to my OB appointment, I felt anxious and excited. Could it be possible that I could be pregnant so quickly after we decided to try? Would my PMDD or more specifically, current migraine, have any effects on my pregnancy? I just spoke out loud, and said if there was anyone in there (growing inside of me), then they already likely knew what the last month had been like, if not more. I explained that while I knew I was ready to welcome them, I was more afraid of physically, how I'd be able to cope with a migraine of this degree and pregnancy. I poured my heart out as if I was writing in a journal. I vocalized my fear, my excitement and joy at the possibility of welcoming a little one. It was then that I made the declaration that if I was indeed pregnant, I would choose to walk through whatever came my way for both of us.

The day I received the confirmation from my OB that my blood test showed that I was indeed pregnant, I was with a doula client doing a few exercises during early labor. They had no idea that there was even a possibility that I was pregnant. In fact, there were only a handful of people that did for that reason. It had been a good day. That morning, I'd gotten up, made breakfast and a smoothie, gone through a few meetings, taken a nap, and went to meet with this family in person. I left their home floating on clouds. I remember sitting in the car and just laughing because there was a whirlwind of thoughts in my mind. At least now there could be no question, I was pregnant, and we had to get to this little one's birthday safely.

The coming weeks meant a few more announcements and searching for a midwife. Unfortunately, it also meant a few more days where I had to reframe how I felt about them. Bad days became days where I needed to care for my body. There were still days that were more difficult than others, but knowing that I needed to push through to meet my end goal gave me the strength to not only get up, but also realize that getting up may look different than what I thought. That has been a lesson that I have had to continuously learn. Some days getting up looks like everything on my to-do list gets done and other days getting up means giving myself the kindness and the grace to rest. The start of 2024 marks three years that I was clued into what was awaiting me a few short months later - not only my son, but an entirely new way of living. A life where every day, I wake up and face what the day may bring, whether it is pushing the gas or hitting the brakes when needed. Chronic pain and illness shapes the way that you look at life, but I choose to embrace the changes it brings. I have to pace my work day which allows me to be very intentional with my time and energy. I know there are going to be some days where I may not be able to operate with 100% strength, but I ensure that I surround myself in peace and love.

My mothering journey has seen multiple feats, and while it is easy to compare myself to others or allow imposter syndrome to win, I am a part of this amazing tribe of women all around the world who choose to get up every day and get it done.

To my Wiggle, may you always know the impact you have had on my life. I waited my entire life for you. I prayed for you, I fought for you, and I will always stand with you. May you continue to grow in life, in health, and in love.

Lare Ngofa is a passionate Health Educator and Doula currently residing in Maryland, though she will always and forever remain a Georgia girl at heart. With a deep devotion to promoting holistic well-being, she founded The Harmony Doula, where they empower individuals and families through education and support during their prenatal, birthing, and postpartum journeys.

Lare finds immense joy in exploring new culinary delights and engaging in unique experiences. As a firm believer in the importance of embracing life's adventures, she actively encourages her son to discover and appreciate the world around us with him by her side. Living with PMDD and migraines has taught her the value of a balanced lifestyle. As a result, she has adopted a 'work hard, rest harder' mentality recognizing the significance of self-care and self-compassion. Through her personal experiences, she strives to normalize discussions around mental health and create safe spaces for open dialogue. With a commitment to empowerment, education, and well-being, she aims to make a positive impact on the lives of those she serves.

Thank You to My Pre-Order Supporters!

Camille Christmas

Your Christmas Crew
https://yourchristmascrew.com
Facebook:
https://www.facebook.com/104467205356774
Instagram: www.instagram.com/yourchristmascrew

Type One-der Woman
Treina Owen

I was born at MCV Hospital in Richmond, VA on July 20, 1979. I grew up as a "Navy Brat." We moved all the time; I even lived in Guantanimo Bay (Gitmo), Cuba. Short, skinny, and dark tanned skin is all I remember, because we were always stationed somewhere in the heat and scorching hot sun. However, when we were stationed in Florida, and my parents were still married, I remember this picture of a chubby dark tanned girl on a Slip-N-Slide, posing with a permed mushroom hairstyle, soaked by the water. Behind my smile was a sad, afraid, mentally, verbally, physically abused little girl who was always being picked on for being just that - chubby, dark tanned skin, oh, and big lipped. After growing up in middle school and enduring some of the most horrific life experiences NO CHILD should ever have to endure, including child rape and molestation by one person, I remember yet another picture of myself taken in 1992. Fake smile, perm-damaged hair in an updo, hands on my hips, wearing an expensive dress that was solid white on the top half and flared out lace on the bottom half. I remember it was 1992 because of the photo's backdrop and my parents were divorced at that time. I was so skinny. Did I lose all that weight because I wasn't being fed properly? Did I lose all that weight because I was on the track team running relay races, jumping hurdles, and throwing shot put? Did I lose all that weight because I also spent many hours practicing my tenor sax so I could keep my 1st chair spot? Did I lose all that weight because I was sad when the chorus teacher said I couldn't take her class because I couldn't sing? Did I lose that weight because I had Type One Diabetes (T1D) (back then they called it Juvenile Diabetes) and just didn't know it? Did the abuse I was enduring cause me to "get" T1D?

Why now, as an adult, am I wondering if I had T1D as a child? In hindsight, it seems like all my paternal side of the family had diabetes and took insulin for it. I remember seeing them check their blood sugars with their meters and inject insulin with syringes. No one on my paternal side ever checked me, nor my siblings, with their meters. Did they know the signs and symptoms to look for in a child? Did they see my weight gain and sudden weight loss or anything else? Did they care? All I know is when God made a way for my brother and I to finally be reunited with our mom, after the system failed us, we were FREE, LOVED, and SAFE!

Let's jump to my last couple of years in high school. I became pregnant in February 1996 and had my first child in November. Being a teenager and pregnant was already hard enough, but being a pregnant teenager with gestational diabetes was the worst! At the time, my mom didn't really know what ALL of this was going to mean, but she took care of it all. She never relied on any government assistance to take care of my brother and me, nor my baby. It was always my mom and granny who took care of us. Mom worked so many jobs so that I didn't have to rely on government assistance for my daughter either. Her insurance wasn't the greatest, thinking back on it now, because I had this "quack" doctor, who still practices to this day, who treated my gestational diabetes. After birth, he came in and didn't even check my glucose (sugar) levels. I remember him saying, "You don't need to see me anymore. You no longer need to take insulin." No test. No bloodwork. No urine sample. No finger pricks. Guess what I did after settling down at home after being discharged from the hospital? I threw out every diabetes supply, meter, and insulin I had—so I thought.

In April 1997, I went on my senior class field trip. We went to Florida and had acted a FOOL at Disney, Epcot, and Daytona Beach. The teachers specifically told us when we went on that trip, no tattoos and no piercings. Well, this French man on the Daytona boardwalk had a tattoo and piercing shop. He told me if I told him I was 18, then I was 18, with no ID, and he gave me an eyebrow piercing. I wasn't 18. The teachers on the trip saw it. I lied and said I got it before the trip. When we returned home, my mom saw it and she was mad.

I came back from that senior trip "sick as a dog!" I was always urinating, sick to my stomach, thirsty, and sleepy. Not only that, months later, it was near graduation time and that eyebrow ring was infected. My skin was so swollen and full of infection I couldn't even unscrew the ball to take the eyebrow ring out! One morning, I woke up with that bloody eyebrow ring on my pillow, because not only was it fake gold, but I was still T1D and didn't know it! Did my mom and granny see the signs and symptoms? Did they care? Yes! Those diabetes supplies I thought I threw out, well, we found my old meter and test strips and tested my sugar. It was so high there was no number on the meter! Just HIGH. Did I have diabetes from November 1996-April 1997 and just didn't know it? Did my high sugars cause my eyebrow infection? I was, later, officially diagnosed as a Type One Diabetic. A teenager. A mother. Feeling like life wasn't fair. I wanted to eat and drink what I wanted and live life like my friends. I don't remember seeing anyone in school like me pricking their finger to test their sugar before each meal and pulling out a syringe to shoot themselves in the stomach with insulin. To this day, I still have a permanent scar on my left eyebrow from where that piercing was. How ironic that it's above the same eye that I have been permanently blind in since 2013, due to diabetic retinopathy. In retrospect, I guess that infected eyebrow ring saved my life.

While the late, great Prince was partying like it's 1999, May 21, 1999, I had to make the decision to have a "late-term abortion" and give birth to my second child. My son. I was almost six months pregnant when I delivered him. At four months pregnant, I went to the restroom at work. As soon as I came back to my desk I "peed" on myself. A co-worker took me to the hospital, which wasn't far. I was leaking amniotic fluid from an unknown source and for an unknown reason. I kept being told you are diabetic and you could die of an infection. Who would take care of my daughter? My unborn son could die because my amniotic fluid would build up, then leak out again. I was told he could eventually die if I had no fluid. I had to make the decision to induce labor and have my child before I officially turned six months pregnant. If I waited until then, they would be liable to save him. If I waited, I could die. I didn't want to leave my daughter without her mother. I didn't want my son to be born prematurely and have tubes, IVs, needles in and out of his body, and living in an incubator until he reached full-term. Doctors told me they couldn't even guarantee that he would survive that. I didn't want him to die in my womb. I didn't want him to suffer outside the womb. I didn't want him growing up with all the horrible health issues and special needs they said he would have. I gave birth to my son on May 21, 1999 and buried him a few days later, with my best friend, Johnell, helping me with all the arrangements. I didn't know God, nor did I believe in Him to perform a miracle, nor did I feel God loved me. If I had known and believed in God then, maybe I wouldn't have listened to the doctors. Maybe I would've prayed more, activated faith, and trusted God for a miracle. Maybe I would've listened to the visitors I had from the United Methodist Church while I was in the hospital making the decision to induce labor. Maybe my son would still be alive. He didn't pass away until sometime after I gave birth. I always felt his movements and kicks. I always wondered who my first son would've grown up to be. I have never gotten over the fact that I didn't give God a try. I was selfish and didn't want my child to grow up sick. I never got over the fact that I killed my son. They said all of this happened *because of my T1D,* but I blamed myself. I carried the guilt of the loss of my son.

One day after visiting the funeral home while making my son's funeral arrangements, I went and got my tongue pierced. I didn't even want to be numbed. I just wanted to feel pain. I couldn't kill myself. I still had a daughter at home who needed me. From then on, I swore I would never have any more children. I was done. But I went on to have another child and had tubal ligation before I left the hospital. She was born with very low blood sugar and had to stay in the NICU for a week. Why—*because of my T1D.* All of the large amounts of concentrated insulin I took caused her to have low blood sugar! Ironically, at the age of five, she was diagnosed with T1D. Another week-long stay in the hospital, IVs, syringes, insulin, and more. While crying out to God for my child, all I could do was think, "what did I do to her?"

All my children are reasons that I continue to live; however, there was a time when I was single with two young daughters and living on my own that I didn't want to live. It was Easter, but also around my younger daughter's birthday. I purposely didn't take any insulin that entire weekend. I had "diabetes burnout." Tired of syringes, tired of medical bills, tired of insulin, tired of living, feeling like I should be able to eat and drink anything I wanted, tired of feeling alone and that no one would ever want me, just tired of life.

> *I almost let go, I felt like I just couldn't take life anymore. My problems had me bound. Depression weighed me down, but God held me close so I wouldn't let go. God's mercy kept me so I wouldn't let go.*

The lyrics to that powerful song by Kurt Carr are what kept me, along with my prayer warrior friend, Crystal, by my side. The God of a second, third, fourth, fifth, and infinite chances KEPT ME so I would still be here for my children, help someone through my experiences, and to one day see a cure for T1D! I would be nowhere without God, my support, and especially my husband, Anson. Just when I didn't think someone would love and accept me for being an unhealthy Type One Diabetic with two children, God laughed, and said I have someone for you!

It was always in my head, since I had my tubes tied, that I wouldn't have any more children so whoever

God sent me had better have his own. Well, Anson didn't and was ok with me not having anymore! We discussed fostering and adopting. We met on Facebook because my best friend was getting married and we both were in the wedding. Let him tell it, I stalked him because I messaged him first. I was just letting it be known that others were asking about him, but I wasn't having that! We officially met in person at a "Fire on Fridays" service at St. Paul's Baptist Church on November 28, 2008. He knew and didn't care about what I was worried about—not being accepted. Of course I had to do a background check on this man who wanted me, a single woman with two daughters. I trusted no one. We were engaged on January 6, 2009 and married by March 12, 2009 at the Justice of the Peace and still went on with the wedding we were already planning for on July 18, 2009. That wedding was probably the most free and beautiful I felt, despite T1D. I walked down the aisle with sight in both eyes and even had in eye contacts. I was able to strap an insulin pen under my wedding dress, free of tubing, beeping, and alarms that I have now with an insulin pump! We've been #theowenfam ever since. My husband even adopted my daughters in 2016!

God continued to laugh, not at us, but at the "they" that I've been referring to, who said this and that would or wouldn't happen *because of my T1D.* HE blessed us in 2011 with our son after two years of getting my tubes UNTIED! The pregnancy wasn't easy and my complications during and after tested our marriage for sure! God kept us when Anson's job fired him for being there for me while I was in the hospital for an entire month before they did an emergency C-section, a month before my due date. I had high protein spilling from my kidneys, high blood pressure, carpal tunnel, preeclampsia, and more *because of my T1D*.

Please note: My T1D is not everyone else's T1D, so everyone's pregnancy will be different and can be successful! Don't let "them" tell you that you can't have a baby when you are T1D.

I always asked God, and Anson, how I could stay at home with our son and not work. Our daughters were always watched by my granny, but I really wanted to stay home with our son and be more active in the girls' school as a volunteer. Be careful what you ask God for! I started noticing a change in my eyes in 2012. I got this cloud over my left eye while traveling to a meeting one day. Before that, I thought one time I couldn't see well at night because it was rainy and dark. I had my eyes checked out by my optometrist and she referred me to go immediately to my retina doctor and that is when I was diagnosed with retina detachment in my left eye. I had two vitrectomy surgeries to try and reattach the retina that failed. My right eye had to have an emergency surgery during the last surgery on my left eye. I have no peripheral vision in the partially blind eye and the laser surgery that I've had is maintaining my vision and preventing my hemorrhages behind my eye from causing complete blindness.

What does it feel like to view the world as if you were me? I have constant anxiety and panic attacks, because I can't see anything coming. Cover your left eye and look straight ahead or turn your whole body. That's how I see the world. However, in my seeing eye, I may see broken lines, black spots, or blurriness, or even a kaleidoscope of colors when I'm having an ocular migraine. After years of yearly eye exams, my optometrist said I had a cataract in my blind eye the size of the entire brown of my eye. I prayed and thought I heard God tell me to see about getting it removed to perhaps be able to see again. I did that and one specialist operated and failed, leaving the brown of my eye wide open exposing the white of that cataract. I remember being in church and directing the children's choir and the children being scared to look at me because of my eye. I felt disgusting. It would be a while after various eye drops and waiting for my eye pressure to go down would another specialist at another practice operate to remove the cataract. I felt every pain of that surgery so much that I almost jumped off the table. Unfortunately, I still can't see out of my blind eye. Over the years, this eye has gotten so bad that I'm losing the eye muscle because it has nothing to focus on, not even a light shining on it in the darkness. I hate even taking pictures now. I have to retake them so many times in order to get a "good one" that somewhat shows both eyes in the same direction.

Despite this discouraging ordeal, my advice is to still take the picture. You never know when it may be the last you take with a loved one.

I've been blessed to be at home to be there with my children and even to take care of other children when needed, including being foster parents to many babies since 2020. Still, in spite of me being a great mom, guilt always sinks in. Why? B*ecause of my T1D*, two out of three of my children have T1D. In addition to our youngest daughter, our son was diagnosed with T1D at age eight. This gave our family an extra push to fight for a cure for T1D and spread awareness, especially in the black community. We have been involved with JDRF since Kamryn (our youngest daughter) was six years old and at each gala, walk, or meet up, she'd feel alone because she never saw any black girls her age at these events. There's also always a misconception that eating too much sugar and no exercise causes T1D, which is untrue. There is no cure for this autoimmune disease and this is why #theowenfam continuously fundraises for the research that has provided improved treatments to survive daily and that will one day find us all cures!

Imagine sometimes dreading hugging your loved ones, holding your husband's hand, your newborn baby's car seat almost falling out of your hand with them in it, not being able to open a bottle of water, insomnia due to pain, feelings of worthlessness and inadequacy, and feeling ugly. Why am I here on this earth? Why did God put me through so much? When will I get a break? I have realized that through all of the pains and complications that I live with daily, people don't see that my chronic illness isn't being faked. I am more than likely faking it to make it and to be an example to those around me that if I can do it, you can do it too! I joke with my husband and kids all the time when life starts life-ing to "never give up and never quit, 'cause you're too legit to quit," in the words of MC Hammer. So, I must be too legit to quit too—it just might take me longer! I still cut my husband and sons' hair. I do my daughters' hair and mine sometimes. I still create with my Cricut, glue gun, and maybe even a hair needle. I home-schooled Karson before he entered preschool and I'm currently teaching our won-da twinz at home now and much more! Through the things I am going through that "they" say are caused by *MY* T1D: multiple trigger finger surgeries, carpal tunnel surgeries, diabetic neuropathy nerve pains, MRIs, EMGs, Botox injections for spinal stenosis pains, epidural injections in the spine, my spinal stenosis surgery to replace discs in my spine so I won't be paralyzed (which I have two more discs that need surgery now), multiple prescriptions to treat my T1D, pain meds, anxiety/depression meds, I feel like Pastor Shirley Caesar—"I got pills, insulin, test strips, meters, CGMs, insulin pumps, YOU NAME IT!" Funny, but not funny! Only I can laugh at my pain and at myself!

My 44 years of life have not been easy, nor has this T1D journey. With God, true friends, and my family, I

GET UP! I still get up and do what needs to be done in whatever pace I may need to that day! I am a wife and mother to three biological children, and twin toddler boys from my heart (that we are praying and believing in God to adopt)! I have a purpose to GET UP! I trust in God to GET UP! I believe in GOD to GET UP! My help comes from GOD to GET UP! Love from God, family and framily lifted me, even when I didn't and don't love myself. My purpose in my T1D fight is to be a Type One-der Woman! The woman who GETS UP and advocates, spreads awareness, finds resources, and educates through my pains and personal experiences with T1D and helps others to do the same! I give God all the credit! T1D or diabetes in general is not as serious to some until it hits them and then I get the texts or inboxes. I am grateful to God I can be there for others. I know, and so do my children with T1D, what it's like to not have support or anyone that looks like you when first diagnosed with T1D. I am the Type One-der Woman who is helping to make sure my children do better with their T1D so they won't have to go through what I went through, are able to advocate for themselves in school and no matter what else life may bring, and be kind and supportive to others when they can. All disabilities aren't visible. You never know what someone is going through. Be the example someone needs so they can GET UP even when they don't feel like it!

Family and FRamily, I love you. Thank you to anyone who's ever loved me and believed in me even when I haven't always loved or believed in myself. To those we've lost, you remain in our hearts. Continue to sleep until Jesus returns.

Treina Owen is from Richmond, VA. She is a wife to Anson Owen, mother to Kyra, Kamryn, Karson, and the Won-Da Twinz, and Tu-Tu to Gabriel. Treina is a passionate person who dedicates her time to fostering children in need, advocating for a cure for diabetes through JDRF initiatives, and indulging in creative, inspirational projects in her spare time. Through the years, she's maintained several leadership roles both in church and in the community. She loves God and owes any accomplishment, seen or unseen, to Him.

Keep in touch with Treina by visiting https://linktr.ee/T1DTreina.

Thank You to My Pre-Order Supporters!

Nuri Anderson

Ariel Brown

Pumped 4 My Journey

www.pumped4myjourney.com

Instagram: Pumped 4 My Journey

CJ Walker

The Genetic Diabetic

www.thegeneticdiabeticblog.com

Facebook: @thegeneticdiabeticblog

Instagram: @thegeneticdiabeticblog

LinkedIn:
https://www.linkedin.com/in/thegeneticdiabetic

Kylene Redmond

Blackdiabetic Girl

Blackdiabeticgirl.com

Instagram: @blackdiabeticgirl

Johnnelle Mayo

Nelles Wreaths

Facebook: Nelles Wreaths

Instagram: @leolioness85

Valerie Travers

Consultancy LLC

Vicki Williams

Facebook: Vicki Fields Williams

Instagram: @Runvicki

Karson Owen

Karson Owen - K.O. a Kure for T1D, T1D Warrior, 2023-2025 JDRF Children's Congress Delegate, JDRF Youth Ambassador

www2.jdrf.org/goto/Koakurefort1d

Instagram: @karsonskicksandthings

Anson Owen

Thesuperhusbaedad

https://linktr.ee/thesuperhusbaedad

Facebook: Thesuperhusbaedad

Instagram: Thesuperhusbaedad

Kamryn Owen

Just Face It Artistry

Instagram: @justfaceitartistry

Kyra Owen

MyKDreamzBeauty

Instagram: @mykdreamzbeauty

Lorraine Edwards

A SINGLE Mission

asinglemission.com

Facebook: @asinglemission

Instagram: @asinglemission

LinkedIn: https://www.linkedin.com/in/lorraine-edwards-msw-asinglemission/

Roshonda Ballard

Facebook: @Roshonda Tabb Ballard

Instagram: @gratefulro27

Donna Page

Dancing with Mama D

https://www.tiktok.com/@dwmdrva?_t=8jilaumXI7y&_r=1

Facebook: @dancingwithmamad

Instagram: @dwmd.rva

Tyrina Bridges

Bridges Is Poppin' LLC (Balloon Decor Service)

Facebook: @bridges.is.poppinllc

Instagram: @bridges_is_poppin

Morgan Carey

Love to Life Coaching, LLC /Love to Juice

www.Lovetolifecoach.com

Facebook: EmjayCee

Instagram: @llcoach_morgan

LinkedIn: https://www.linkedin.com/in/morgan-carey-mshrm-shrm-cp-47ba8676?utm_source=share&utm_campaign=share_via&utm_content=profile&utm_medium=ios_app

Quenia Herrera

Every Step I Take
Karen Robinson

"But he was wounded for our transgressions, he was bruised for our iniquities: the chastisement of our peace was upon him; and with his stripes we are healed." Isaiah 53:5

What does a day look like in the life of me - a person with several medical challenges? Anxiety and depression, lots of tears, and restricted mobility. I'm not able to just jump out of bed and start walking. My current state of health requires me to sit and carefully pace myself so I don't fall. I have to consciously think about the next step that I'm going to take as I walk because at any moment, my back can go out and I'll be down on the floor! There have been so many countless nights that my children had to help me up the stairs to the bedroom, to the bathroom, and even to the car.

The summer of 2001 is when my medical complications all began. The transition was tough. The most difficult part about persisting through the challenges was getting up and putting on my mask.

You know, the mask of everything being alright and perfect over here to step out into the eye of the public. The truth is, however, everything was not alright and people had no idea what it took for me to get both feet on the floor on a daily basis. Nevertheless, I continued to get up. With seven children looking to me for guidance, for protection, and love, I had no other option! Everything each child needed and desired, they were looking to me to provide and I was looking to my Lord and Savior for the strength and the ability to provide that to them.

As my medical conditions increased, my ability to function was decreasing. My first diagnosis was hypertension along with Lyme disease and rheumatoid arthritis. I was petrified! It was challenging to tunnel through those diagnoses! Shortly after, anxiety and depression had overtaken me. I felt so lost and worthless. My body was trying to adjust to medication and my anxiety was causing me not to trust the medication. I was told so many things by so many people. Some suggested going holistic and others said stick with the medical doctors' regimen. I despised the medication because it caused so many side effects. But the weight of the whole entire family was upon my shoulders and I had to get up.

I became even more depressed while continuing to deal with my medical challenges. In 2013, I injured my lower spine. I thought it was the end of the world for me. This pain was so overwhelming, I could hardly think straight. To add insult to injury, one doctor in particular thought I was faking my pain. Here I was dealing with hypertension, Lyme disease, rheumatoid arthritis, and this lower back injury with severe pain. What a setback! I didn't think I could survive! I felt helpless and it seemed like I was in a hopeless situation. But little did I know, that wouldn't even be the end of my medical challenges.

In 2016, I was in a car accident. A drunk driver ran the red light and T-boned me. My neck snapped and caused my upper spine to be impinged. This spine injury resulted in me losing even more mobility and caused tremors in my hands. I couldn't hold a coffee cup without spilling its contents or without dropping it altogether. I was told I had to have surgery or one wrong fall and I could be paralyzed. Boy did that increase my anxiety and it also increased my depression! Nevertheless, I had to tunnel through that. I continued to wear a mask of everything being okay. I kept getting up. It was mandatory because so many people depended on me. My mother who had dementia (God rest her soul) was depending on me. My father, a colon cancer survivor, was depending on me. My children were still depending on me. Although I could barely take care of myself, so many were depending on me. I had no one to look to but God! I had to persevere; I had to push through; and I had to show up for them! I had to get up!

My ability to get up would not have been possible without the Lord on my side. Looking back in hindsight, I could have been paralyzed and in a wheelchair. I could've had a stroke due to hypertension and I could've been severely affected by Lyme disease. While chronic pain is the most traumatic of all my illnesses because it can't be seen, physically, I suffer day in and day out with it. It is very invasive and controlling. It disrupts most activities that I try to participate in, and God forbid lifting items. How am I surviving? By the grace of God and a good medication regimen.

People think there is nothing wrong with you because pain is invisible. Pain is inward. Pain is unpredictable. Pain doesn't stand out like other illnesses with visible symptoms. Pain is hidden, so therefore people don't take you seriously when chronic pain is your number one diagnosis. It has taken over my life and I continue to deal with it on a daily basis. I am so thankful that when you look at me I don't look like what I've been through and I don't look like what I'm going through! I've been through the fire and there is no trace of smoke or burn marks on me. If it wasn't for my medication regimen, I wouldn't be able to do half of the things that I can do so I thank God for medical technology. I thank God for the education of the doctors, and I thank God for His grace and His mercy! That combination gives me the ability to get up. It gives me the ability to keep moving one step at a time!

I commend anyone who is dealing with any type of medical challenge but perseveres and pushes themselves to get up! Get up and keep fighting the good fight because God is with us. He is the one who gives us the strength and the ability to keep going in a situation that seems impossible. Although hard, I've had to embrace the fact that my medical conditions do not define me. They are a part of my story, but they do not dictate my worth or potential. With each day, I choose to focus on my strengths, passions, and the boundless possibilities that lie ahead. By honoring my true essence and embracing all that I am, I walk forward with courage, determination, and a profound sense of purpose. I am not limited by my medical conditions; I am empowered by the unwavering love of Jesus Christ and the infinite possibilities that He has in store for me.

Karen Bailey Robinson, a North Carolina native, is a retired housewife by day and an aspiring actor by night. She is the biological mother to a beautiful daughter (Kayla) and two sons (Bautista and Victor

Jr.) and adoptive mother to her two nieces (Tameika and Malaysia). She is an ordained Elder in the Lord's church and she enjoys working for the Lord in any capacity for she is a servant leader at heart. Karen studied Human Service and Drug and Alcohol Counseling at Delaware Technical Community College in Wilmington, Delaware and is currently studying Ministry Leadership at Lancaster Bible College in Philadelphia, PA. In her spare time, she enjoys singing, acting, reading, and spending quality time with her grandchildren. Karen is a co-author of Amazon's Best-Sellers, After the Storm and Resisting Temptation: Overcoming and Surviving Addiction. She currently resides in Philadelphia sharing life with the love of her life, Khalif.

You can connect with her on Facebook at https://www.facebook.com/cherlydine.bailey or by visiting her website at vicmpa.org.

Thank You to My Pre-Order Supporters!

Kayla McRae

B.B.E. Bountiful blessing by Elijah

Facebook: @charlottelove

Instagram: @bigblu2023

Brenda Esaw-Howard

Celebration of Life 2000 Breast Cancer Awareness Program   www.celebrationoflife2000.com

Facebook: @celebrationoflife2000

Instagram: @celebrationoflife2000

LinkedIn: Celebrationoflife2000

Ralph Robinson

Ursula Jones

Prissy Tx Mobile Notary Service

Prissytxnotary.com

Facebook: @Ursulapriscillajones

Instagram: @prissyjvlogs

Mary Williams

J& K Financial Services

Weakness As My Greatest Strength
Chazley Williams

Each time he said, "My grace is all you need. My power works best in weakness. So now I am glad to boast about my weaknesses, so that the power of Christ can work through me."-**II Corinthians 12:9 NLT**

Diabetes is a debilitating disease that can alternately affect so many parts of your body if not managed well. The disease runs deep in my family. I witnessed it take the life of my maternal grandmother and aunt and I see the physical debilitating effects it is currently having on my mother. I have always feared it, but no matter my efforts to prevent it, I could not escape it. From Chronic Kidney Disease, hearing loss, skin issues, gastric issues, and a recent seizure, diabetes has tried to control and take my life many times, but God has kept me.

I'm not sure when I became a diabetic, but I have been on diabetes medication for at least ten years. Diabetes does not care how old, how big, or how small you are. It doesn't care about your diet or lifestyle. Sometimes, becoming a diabetic is inevitable due to genetics or dietary history. I remember having moments in high school when I felt weak. My mom would check my blood sugar with a finger stick glucometer. As I matriculated on to college, there were a few times when I felt like my blood sugar was possibly dropping. However, instead of getting myself checked out or looking more into these issues, I swept them under the rug as I didn't want anything else to deal with. I was already battling enough health issues.

While spending time at a street festival in DC with friends in the summer of 2015, I became hot, felt dehydrated, nauseous, and vomited most of the day. Talk about embarrassing. I walked through the festival vomiting at every stop until my friends finally managed to get me through the crowd. Eventually, I went to the doctor and was told my creatinine level (a measure of how your kidneys filter waste from your blood) was low and a kidney biopsy was recommended. After getting the kidney biopsy, I was told that I had Stage 2b kidney disease which meant my kidneys had mild damage and were less able to filter waste and fluid out of my blood. This was a result of being a diabetic and having high blood pressure issues in the past. Nevertheless, I was told that if I took my high blood pressure medication and diabetic medication, I should be fine for years to come.

Unfortunately, I also found out around the same time that my mother had to have cancerous cells removed from her kidney that year. That also resulted in her having kidney disease as she had been an insulin dependent diabetic for over 30 years. As time progressed, I would continue to find out, "the apple really didn't fall too far from the tree" in my case.

Fast forward to May 2018, I got married to my amazing husband, Brandon, but tragically lost my aunt (my mother's only living sister) from diabetes complications in October 2018. Keep that in mind as most of us know that stress and trauma can destroy the body in many ways. Some of us harbor trauma in our minds and some in our bodies. In my case, I believe most of my life stressors were harbored in my physical health. My kidneys had been doing alright until January 2019 when I was hospitalized for complications from a high dosage of prednisone that I was prescribed for a sinus infection. Doctors noticed then that my kidney function was getting worse due to the high dose of prednisone elevating my glucose quickly. With medical attention, my glucose came down, but alternatively, my kidneys suffered. I started to notice that my urine was changing, my feet were beginning to swell, and I gained a lot of weight. Around July 2019, I went to see my Nephrologist and he said my kidney function was in stage 4 and I needed to start thinking about treatment options - dialysis or a kidney transplant.

During this time, my mom was also beginning to experience health issues again. This time, with complications from her diabetes. After intense operations and progressing Vascular Dementia, my sister and I had to alternatively move her out of her home and into a long-term care nursing home.

As my feet continued to swell to the point of barely being able to put shoes on, I subsequently became sicker and sicker. My nephrologist told me in August I was progressing to stage 5, which is end stage kidney failure. We went through the process of being added to the kidney transplant list at VCU/MCV hospital and Duke University Medical Center, a process that would include hours of uncomfortable testing and a donor wait that was likely to take up to five years.

In denial and determined my new diagnosis was a lie, I visited a holistic doctor to see what I could do to reverse my diagnosis. I was advised to go vegan, which my husband and I did for almost two months. This rapid decline was rare for a 30-year-old. Still, it was a reality that I had to face.

People tend to ask me why I was in denial and didn't just accept the diagnosis. For me, it was different. An unplanned child born to older parents, my mom had complications during her delivery with me. I came out of the wound being somewhat different. I was born with a brachial plexus injury (left shoulder, arm and hand paralyzed) and was used to going to doctors and having surgeries. I thought I left that life in the past. I hoped to finally live a somewhat normal life. In fact, I had prayed most of my life for a normal life.

As I continued to pray that I would not have to go on kidney dialysis, I attended a Kidney Smart class to learn more about kidney disease treatments that my doctor recommended. During the class, I couldn't focus because my body was experiencing so much weakness and pain and I felt nauseous. My husband took me to the hospital immediately after the class and I was put on emergency kidney dialysis in the hospital. I was in the hospital for a week getting dialysis, medication, and had a dialysis port installed to receive peritoneal dialysis once released.

During that exact same time, my mom was also in the hospital about to go into a life-changing surgery back home in Danville, VA, about two and a half hours from me in Richmond, VA. I couldn't be with her and she couldn't be with me. My biggest supporter, the person who always made sure I was safe, couldn't be with me. All I could do was pray for God to cover us both. My sister went to be with mom and my husband was with me.

After my husband and a best friend underwent weeks of training at a DaVita Dialysis Center with me, I started peritoneal dialysis from October 2019 until October 2020. Peritoneal dialysis is typically done at home eight hours a day using a dialysis machine that is connected to your abdomen to remove toxins in those with kidney failure. My husband and I had to make sure our new house, which we had only been in a year, was deemed safe for dialysis. The house had to always be clean and a nurse had to come in and make sure it was safe. We had to basically turn one of our bedrooms into a medical supply closet and large bags of fluid were shipped to my house every few weeks. For eight hours, seven days a week, my husband hooked me up to the dialysis machine since I couldn't do it due to my brachial plexus injury of my left arm. I went from being a child who felt like a burden (because I had to always ask for help) to an adult who felt like one. Those who know me know that asking for help is the hardest thing for me to do. Throughout the sleepless nights, weight gain, weight loss, hair loss, stress, and self-esteem issues, I didn't think I could make it, but here I am. I still woke up every day and went to work and tried to find a new normal. I even eventually returned to my online master's degree program, which I had to pause a few times from when I initially went on dialysis as I navigated these uncharted waters.

While I was in my master's program, I told my professor that it was too much for me to be in school during that time and I needed to take a break. Thankfully, I was in an online program, so I never had to physically go to class. My professor was very understanding. He wished me well and told me that not only did he have a friend who had received a transplant, but also that he was planning to be an organ donor for someone one day as well. I asked him to pray for me as I didn't have a donor and was hoping I could return to school some day.

In July 2020, I decided it was time I go back to school despite being on dialysis, as I was now getting the hang of my routine. This would be my new normal. When I returned to school I registered for the same class, which was taught by the same professor as before. About a week into my course, I received an email from my professor that he wanted to speak to me. When we spoke, he asked if I had found a kidney donor yet and I advised him that I had not. He let me know that he had been tested and cleared to be a donor for a child that lived in the area, but the child had a few options. My professor then told me he was available to be my kidney donor if we were matched. Within a few weeks he was tested and we were a match! I had found my kidney donor! On November 9, 2020, I met my professor and his wife for the first time in-person before the operation the next day, November 10, 2020.

January 2021, I decided to go back and finish what I started. I graduated with my Master's in Education in May 2022. After starting and stopping many times, I was determined to never give up. That degree, in a strange twist of fate, ended up saving my life.

What most people do not understand, however, is that a kidney transplant is not a cure, though it does give you a better lifestyle than dialysis. Yes, I am so grateful for my gift of life, but I am also cautious as I still have many health issues to monitor. I am tied to transplant medications for life, a weakened immune system, consistent blood work and hospital visits. After my transplant, I immediately began taking 12 pills a day, two of which were new diabetic medications as my diabetes got worse after my transplant from the medication. I am now an insulin dependent diabetic, permanently on insulin three times a day, but I am grateful to even still be here.

In January 2023, the week before my birthday, my sister and I were taking our monthly drive to Danville to visit my mom. As my sister was talking to me while driving, my body began twitching and I blacked out. The next thing I recall was waking up in an ambulance talking to an EMT about the illnesses I have and the fact that I have three kidneys in my body. I ended up going to two hospitals, having multiple tests done, and eventually being admitted to VCU/MCV ICU for a week. I was diagnosed with diabetic ketoacidosis and had a seizure from my body reacting to medication that I began taking after my transplant. I was released on my 34th birthday.

How Am I Healing?

Three things come to mind with my healing process: God, rest, and therapy.

God

I was raised in a small, black southern Baptist church and trained to learn old black church hymns by heart. I knew the song "Jesus Loves Me" by age five, *though I am weak, but he is strong…* learned the 23rd Psalms by age eight. I was raised to have faith in God no matter what, pray no matter what, praise no matter what. With all of that, I still managed to stray away from God and church many times. Asked God why many times. Felt like a burden so many times. Eventually, I fell into a depression. How can God allow a 30-year-old to go through all of this and just when it looks like my life is finally coming together? Why must my husband deal with this? He doesn't deserve this.

Like Paul in Corinthians, I begged God three times to take this handicap away!

But through it all, God never left my side. I had to remember that the same God who saved me so many times before, who healed me many times before, would do it again. By His stripes, I am healed. I have been given a gift of life with my kidney donation. God is giving me the opportunity to inspire someone else to keep going.

There are days when I sit in hospitals, labs or at home, giving myself insulin or getting blood drawn. I sing to myself, "*the blood that gives me strength from day to day...it will never lose its power.*" Singing those old hymns that used to bore me as a child are what's healing me as an adult. God is healing me. We must stop trying to figure out the plan and leave it to God.

Rest

As mentioned, stress can have many negative effects on our body. I know now that I could have prevented some of my health complications if I had just sat down and rested. I never learned anything about self-care growing up. Most of my adulthood I've worked multiple jobs. I also used work as a distraction to not have to worry about what was going on in my life. I was taught to stay busy and you won't have time to worry.

It took being 30 and almost losing my life to prioritize rest and stillness. There is no way to hear God clearly if you don't sit down, get still, and rest. I had to "take my cape off" and learn that it is okay to be strong and weak, simultaneously.

Therapy

Being raised by an old school black mother, therapy was unheard of. I held onto so much heartache and grief over the years from my own disabilities to watching my dad have a heart attack and die when I was four to now watching my mom mentally deteriorate. Just like stress, grief and trauma can hold a weight on your body, that if you do not release, will tear you apart.

However, I initially decided to go to therapy before I got married to deal with some of my "Daddy issues", then later ended up digging into some of my trauma and grief that have deeply helped me with my mental healing, which is also healing me physically. I am finally incorporating the right tools to change how I think about myself, loving and taking care of myself.

Through God, Rest and Therapy, I am getting up and not giving up.

Chazley Williams is from Danville, Virginia and is a kidney transplant survivor living with diabetes. She believes, "I have kidney disease; it doesn't have me." Chazley is an educator, caregiver, writer, and visionary who aims to continue to inspire others. Chazley is an advocate for disability rights, health, and diversity issues. She currently resides in Richmond, VA with her devoted husband, Brandon.

Thank You to My Pre-Order Supporters!

Tiffany Winfield

Selah74

Selah74.com

Facebook: @Selah74

Instagram: @Selah_74_

Fonda Neal

Fonda Neal Natural Health, LLC

www.fondanealnaturalhealth.com

Facebook: @FondaMikellHeathNeal

Tamara Dias

Good Soil Education

www.begoodsoil.com

Facebook: @drtamarawdias

Instagram: @drtamarawdias

LinkedIn.com/in/tamarawdias

Conclusion

As we reach the conclusion of *Girl, Get Up: An Inspirational Guide for Women Living with Autoimmune Disease, Chronic Illness, and Pain*, we are reminded of the profound resilience that resides within each woman who has shared her story within these pages. Their voices, though varied in tone and experience, unite in a powerful chorus of courage, strength, and hope.

Throughout this journey, we have witnessed the raw vulnerability of diagnosis, the relentless struggle against symptoms, and the profound impact of these conditions on every aspect of life. Yet, in the face of adversity, these women have not faltered. They have stood tall, facing each challenge with unwavering determination and grace.

Their stories serve as a beacon of light for all who walk a similar path. They remind us that we are not defined by our illnesses, but by the strength with which we confront them. They inspire us to rise above the limitations imposed upon us and to embrace life with renewed vigor and purpose.

As we close the pages of this book, let us carry with us the lessons of resilience, compassion, and empathy that these women have so generously shared. Let us be reminded that our struggles do not define us, but rather, they shape us into the resilient, compassionate beings that we are meant to be.

To every woman who has bravely shared her story, thank you. Thank you for your courage, your strength, and your unwavering determination to rise above adversity. May your voices continue to echo in the hearts of all who read these pages, inspiring hope, courage, and resilience in the face of life's greatest challenges.

And to every reader who has embarked on this journey with us, may you find solace, strength, and inspiration in the stories of these remarkable women. May you be reminded that no matter how dark the night may seem, there is always hope on the horizon, waiting to guide you towards a brighter tomorrow.

So, dear reader, as you close this book, remember these words: **Girl, Get Up**. Rise above the challenges that life throws your way. Embrace your inner strength, your resilience, and your unwavering determination to overcome. For in the journey of life, it is not the destination that defines us, but the strength with which we face each step along the way.

Girl, Get Up. Your journey is just beginning.

www.ingramcontent.com/pod-product-compliance
Lightning Source LLC
Chambersburg PA
CBHW070252290326
41930CB00041B/2455